LEAD IS
A SILENT
HAZARD

LEAD IS A SILENT HAZARD

RICHARD M. STAPLETON

FOREWORD BY
SENATOR BILL BRADLEY

WALKER AND COMPANY ✹ NEW YORK

First published in the United States of America in 1994 by
Walker Publishing Company, Inc.

Published simultaneously in Canada by Thomas Allen & Son Canada, Limited,
Markham, Ontario

Library of Congress Cataloging-in-Publication Data
Stapleton, Richard M.
Lead is a silent hazard / Richard M. Stapleton ; foreword by
Senator Bill Bradley.
p. cm.
Includes index.
ISBN 0-8027-1303-3. — ISBN 0-8027-7449-0 (pbk.)
1. Lead—Toxicology. 2. Pediatric toxicology. I. Bradley, Bill,
1943– . II. Title.
RA1231.L4S65 1994
615.9'25688—dc20   94-5320
CIP

BOOK DESIGN BY KATY RIEGEL

Printed in the United States of America

2   4   6   8   10   9   7   5   3   1

CONTENTS

ACKNOWLEDGMENTS

There are so many people to thank: George Gibson, my publisher, for his unflagging enthusiasm and support; Jackie Johnson and Vicki Haire, my editors, for their sensitive surgery; Carol Mann, my agent, for going that extra step; the many professionals—professors, doctors, researchers, scientists, health-care providers, environmentalists, and advocates in both private and public sectors—quoted throughout, who gave so generously of their time, expertise, and encouragement; the parents, quoted and referenced, who shared so much—retelling and thereby reliving what for most was a nightmare of guilt, frustration, and helplessness—so that others might learn from their experience; my own family, for their incredible support and understanding those endless long nights and weekends when I was lost to the computer; additional thanks to my wife, Andrea, for reading and rereading draft after draft.

Finally, there is my son Matthew, whose giggle-breaks and interruptions to play "letters" on the computer were a constant reminder of the importance of writing this book; it is to him, with love, that *Lead Is a Silent Hazard* is dedicated.

FOREWORD

Lead is the most critical, most costly environmental health problem that faces our children today. That opinion is shared by the U.S. Environmental Protection Agency, the Centers for Disease Control, and the Department of Health and Human Services. The CDC estimates that up to 10 percent of all children may have an unacceptably high level of lead in their blood, and 10,000 more children are poisoned annually. Yet while lead poisoning can lead to permanent neurological damage and ongoing learning and behavioral problems, it is completely preventable.

The threat to our children from lead exposure is very real. It persists today in our soil, in the air, in our drinking water, and in our homes. It crosses all social, economic, and geographic lines. The most dangerous source of lead poisoning is house dust containing lead-based paint from walls, doorjambs, and window sashes. Most homes built prior to 1978 contain at least some lead-based paint. According to the Department of Housing and Urban Development, about 3.8 million families in the United States with young children live in homes with lead hazards. New research suggests that a health threat exists even at very low exposures. No child is safe from this threat. No parent can afford to remain uninformed.

Our biggest single lead problem in this nation is still a lack of knowledge about lead. *Lead Is a Silent Hazard* will serve as a critical resource for parents interested in protecting their children from this number-one environmental health hazard facing preschoolers. It collects in a single volume the most up-to-date information about the threat from lead, testing and treatment, potential safeguards, and related public efforts.

Addressing this problem in the future will require a concerted effort by legislators and private citizens alike. Parents must do what they can, including having their children tested for lead exposure and ensuring that their homes are safe. I also encourage everyone reading this book to become involved in local and federal efforts to remove the threat. In the past, congressional legislation focused on limiting the growth of the threat and alerting the public to the risks. We also outlawed lead-paint use in housing, stopped burning lead with our gasoline, and prohibited the practice of using lead in drinking-water systems.

More needs to be done. Congress must also address the approximately $10-billion problem of severe lead hazards in our low-income housing stock and day-care centers. In low-income households in urban areas, for example, 68 percent of the black children and 36 percent of the white children are estimated to have unsafe blood-lead levels. I have been working hard in the Congress to address this problem. But it will take all of us working together to make our nation safer from this deadly threat to the most vulnerable among us—our children.

—Senator Bill Bradley

PREFACE

*The modern history of lead poisoning is a
sad tale of inexcusable disregard for
knowledge that has long existed.*

—*Jane S. Lin-Fu*
U.S. Dept. of Health
and Human Services

We learned quite by accident. We had no reason to suspect that our baby was being lead poisoned. His blood test was to have been a postscript to a story I was writing. But he was being poisoned, silently, insideously, under our watchful and loving eyes. And suddenly, we found ourselves living a story I had originally set out to report.

It has been a disquieting experience. I'm of the old school, trained to be the dispassionate reporter, observing at arm's length: What happened? What does that mean? How did that make you feel? Afraid? Angry? Confused? Frustrated? Guilty? The words take on new meaning when you live them. And you will, if your child tests high. You're a parent.

My wife Andrea and I are both seasoned journalists, experienced in gathering information quickly. We set out to learn about lead poisoning, confident we'd quickly track down the silent hazard that was poisoning our son. Yet it took weeks for us to learn the many sources of lead in our lives. It took even longer to learn how to deal with them.

Dr. Lin-Fu must speak of the experts when she laments the disregard of knowledge long held. The deadliness of lead has been known for centuries (Benjamin Franklin wrote a chilling letter on the subject)—but for most of us the information has been a well-kept secret.

You cannot disregard what you do not know. Andrea and I didn't know much.

We learned, though. We learned that no matter where you live, no matter how nice your neighborhood, no matter how expensive your home, if it contains lead-based paint, your child is at risk from lead poisoning. Lead poisoning has been and still is the scourge of the slums: Fully 40 percent of the children born in the poorest sections of our cities suffer low-level lead poisoning. However, the children at greatest risk of *acute* lead poisoning are kids whose parents have the resources to buy and renovate beautiful older homes.

We learned that lead lurks in countless corners: It can be in the watercooler at school, on the windowsills at your day-care center, or in the dirt in your own backyard. It is in lead crystal and the seals on fine wines, in your dishes and coffee mugs, in crayons and on toys. It may even be in the calcium supplements you take in the name of good nutrition.

The more we learned, the madder we got. Mad because we realized that we had poisoned our precious child. Not out of disregard, but out of ignorance. Out of other's disregard for our need to know.

In the end, we were lucky. By getting an early warning, and by aggressively working to eliminate the sources of lead, we were able to prevent serious long-term damage. Lead is ubiquitous, and its effects are cumulative. Every child who is exposed to lead is almost certainly exposed to more than one source of lead. You need to identify and deal with each and every path of contamination if you're to fully protect your child, but we discovered that many sources can be easily eliminated or avoided—even the most serious problems sometimes have reasonable, relatively inexpensive solutions. The key is having good information.

This book will arm you, as a parent, with the information you need to protect your child from lead poisoning. My hope is that by helping you deal with the practical problems, it will also help you deal with the emotional ones; the latter can be as overwhelming as the former. My other hope is that this book will alarm and anger you to the point that you take some action—a letter, an E-mail message, a contribution—to help raise the national awareness of our legacy of lead.

While our first concern as parents must be the protection of our own children, we cannot ignore America's collective cultural loss. Lead poisoning squanders the intelligence potential of a cross-section of our country. We are filling entire school systems with children handicapped by hyperactivity and hobbled by attention disorders, yet we wonder why we can't educate them.

LEAD IS A SILENT HAZARD

1

THE SILENT HAZARD

"*Matthew has an elevated lead level.*"

THE NEWS HIT like a punch in the stomach. I was producing a daily environmental broadcast for CBS News and had just finished researching a story about the effects of childhood lead poisoning; I knew what an elevated lead level could mean. Lead poisoning is far and away the greatest environmental threat our children face. The U.S. Environmental Protection Agency estimates that one of every ten preschoolers suffers from some form of lead poisoning. Even low levels of lead can block an infant's mental development. Lead in a child's system can lower that child's IQ enough to cause a potential genius (my child, of course!) to drop to an average achievement level, and it can leave an average child learning disabled.

Almost as an afterthought, while working on my broadcast, I had asked our pediatrician to test Matthew for lead poisoning. My wife and I expected the results to be another "reflexes okay, weight and length about average" reassurance that everything was normal. But it wasn't. We had an intruder in our home, an invisible thief bent on stealing our baby's brainpower. Our little boy was being silently poisoned.

Our children live, one expert writes, in a world of lead. Matthew certainly did. A do-it-yourself lead-test kit told us that some surface paint in our home contained lead. No surprise, really; almost every house built before 1976 contains at least some lead paint, and ours was built in the 20s. Another test showed our tap water to be a source. Plumbing is a classic source of lead poisoning, and we discovered lead-soldered copper pipes in the house and a solid lead pipe bringing water in from the street.

We had been renovating our new home while Andrea was pregnant with Matthew, and thus she was nagged by a mother's question, "Did I do this to my baby?" She was haunted by the fear that she had unwittingly exposed our unborn baby to this poison even as we worked to ready his new home. We will never know the answer for certain, but we learned that many home renovations where kids are present result in childhood lead poisoning. The risk could have been prevented, had we only known.

SOME BASIC FACTS ABOUT LEAD POISONING

Lead poisoning is the number-one environmental health threat our children face today. We raise our children in homes and yards and a nation contaminated with lead. Lead has no positive value to the human body and has not been shown to be safe at any level. One in ten American children—over 1.7 million kids—have unacceptable levels of lead in their blood, and what is considered acceptable today may be proven unacceptable tomorrow.

The good news is that lead poisoning is totally preventable, and there's a lot you can do yourself to protect your child. Most lead poisoning happens in and around the home. Once you identify the sources of your child's exposure to lead, you can reduce or eliminate them, sometimes with little cost and effort. There are even nutritional steps you can take to keep your child's body from absorbing lead. And certain house-cleaning precautions can reduce the threat of lead-dust poisoning.

The key to preventing lead poisoning is knowledge—knowing what to do and what not to do. For example, deteriorating lead paint in a child's home is hazardous, but removing it improperly can turn the potential for low-level poisoning into the reality of acute lead poisoning.

Children are at special risk because their bodies process lead differently than adults. Children absorb up to 50 percent of the lead they ingest—adults retain only 10 percent. This high retention occurs during the early formative years when the central nervous system, including the brain, is developing. Lead interferes with that development. By the time physical symptoms are evident—headaches, nausea, weakness—significant brain damage has already occurred.

It doesn't take much lead to poison a child. An amount equal to one granule of sugar each day over a period of time will raise a child's blood lead level to 35 μg/dl, high enough to trigger intervention and treatment. According to the Centers for Disease Control (CDC), the threshold for poisoning is just 10 μg/dl (see box, p. 4).

Contact with lead is unavoidable. Nobody is immune. No class, no race, no community, no one. Half of all inner-city children suffer from lead poisoning, yet some of the highest levels of lead poisoning are found in the children of middle- and upper-class families who are renovating expensive homes. Lead poisoning is thought of as an urban problem, but people living in North Carolina and Missouri are finding that the problem is worse out on the farm than it is in the city. Lead is invisible. Tasteless. Odorless. It accumulates in the body; long-term consumption of low levels can be more dangerous than a single ingestion of concentrated lead. Lead attacks the unborn child in the mother's womb, and children remain at special risk at least through age seven. Even at low levels in the blood, lead attacks the child's developing brain. At high levels, lead can kill.

We have had to change our perception of lead poisoning. For years, lead poisoning was seen as an acute disease, affecting a relatively small percentage of the population. Education, regulation, intervention, and treatment have all but eliminated lead poisoning as a killer of children in America. As a result, many people view the whole subject of lead poisoning as a problem of the past.

This notion is reinforced by the fact that average blood-lead levels in America have come down dramatically. In the past 20 years, the federal government has banned the use of lead in paint and in gasoline. The food industry has stopped using lead-soldered cans. In 1976, the average level of lead in our blood was 17 μg/dl; today it is about 4 μg/dl. However, as average blood-lead levels have come down, scientists have been better able to measure the effects of lower-level exposure to lead. We are coming to know lead poisoning to be a much less dangerous disease in terms of its severity—but a much more threatening one in terms of the size and spectrum of the population it affects.

In low-level lead poisoning (10 μg/dl), there are no symptoms and there is no treatment. The only answer is prevention—eliminating sources of lead before the child is further poisoned. In acute lead poisoning (60 μg/dl), there are overt symptoms, and the primary concern

THAT μG/DL TECHNICAL STUFF

Unless you are a scientist, the μg/dl's, ppm's, and ppb's that you will encounter could make your eyes glaze over. Unfortunately, we need to use these units of measure occasionally so we know when we're talking about apples and when we're talking about oranges. Don't try to memorize what they mean; the important thing to know is that 60 apples is more than 10 apples.

μg/dl is used to describe the amount of lead in blood. It's short-hand for micrograms (μg) per deciliter (dl). A microgram is one millionth of a gram, and there are 28 grams in an ounce. A deciliter is a tenth of a liter, equal to about half a cup. You'd get a concentration of 1 μg/dl if you flooded a football field with two feet of water and tossed in one tablespoon of sugar.

ppm, used to measure levels of contamination, stands for parts per million. A big truck overturns and spills one million oranges. Workmen cleaning up the mess discover one apple. That's one part per million.

ppb, used the same way, stands for parts per billion. One hundred trucks overturn and spill one billion oranges. Workmen find one apple. That's one part per billion, which also equals one microgram per deciliter (1 ppb = 1 μg/dl).

AND THEN THERE ARE ALL THOSE ACRONYMS

ATSDR, CDC, EPA, HHS . . . what would government agencies be without acronyms? One thing I do know is that without them, this book would include a lot more pages! Whenever an agency is referred to for the first time, I'll use the full name, along with its acronym. After that, it's alphabet soup. If you forget, you can look it up in appendix A.

is treatment. Common symptoms include headaches, stomachaches, cramps, or vomiting. The child may be tired, cranky, clumsy, or lose interest in playing. Diagnosis can be difficult since those symptoms also occur in any number of childhood maladies.

Low-level lead poisoning reduces intelligence, causes reading and learning disabilities, and has been linked to later failure to graduate from high school and to criminal behavior. It can also cause such behavioral problems as hyperactivity and reduced attention span. Physical effects include low birth weight and size, loss of hearing, and delayed physical development. Signs of possible lead poisoning include delayed developmental milestones like standing, walking, and talking, but by the time these are noted, damage has been done. *A blood lead test is the only reliable way to diagnose lead poisoning.*

There is a lot more to learn about the effects of lead at the lowest levels, but it is becoming clear that lead *at any level* poses a threat to children. As we learn more about the effects of low-level lead poisoning, the so-called action level—the point at which we say a person is lead poisoned—keeps moving down. In the mid-1960s, people weren't considered poisoned until their blood-lead level hit 60 µg/dl. The number was cut in half in 1978, dropped again in 1985, and lowered to the present 10 µg/dl in October 1991.

PRENATAL EXPOSURE TO LEAD

Exposure to lead starts even before conception. The body stores lead. Its half-life (the length of time it takes to reduce the concentration of lead by 50 percent) in blood and soft tissue is about a month. Lead's half-life in bone is some thirteen *years* for adults. (The figure is unknown for children.) In times of stress, including pregnancy, the lead stored in bones is released into the blood stream. Lead easily crosses the placental barrier throughout the gestation period, including the critical period during which the central nervous system is formed.

By reducing lead intake for at least two months prior to conception, the mother-to-be can lower the amount of lead stored in her body. This in turn will reduce the amount of lead her baby is exposed to once she conceives. Reducing exposure to lead while pregnant is especially important because pregnant women absorb much more of the lead they ingest than do other adults.

We learned of the danger of in-utero poisoning long after Matthew was born, after Andrea had seemingly spent her entire pregnancy either

Bone analysis—bones store 95 percent of the lead in an adult body—shows that our early ancestors had virtually no lead in their bodies. Lead is an element; it doesn't break down, burn up, biodegrade, or dissipate. Lead poisoning is the by-product of industry. Researchers studying sediment layers from the bottoms of Swedish lakes have been able to trace lead pollution back 2,600 years, to lead dust released when the ancient Greeks began refining silver. Concentrations of lead pollution peaked 600 years later at the height of the Roman Empire, then faded away for almost two millennium, only to soar again with the advent of the Industrial Revolution in the 1800s. Every microgram of lead that has been released into the environment is still there. And there's a lot of it.

The Agency for Toxic Substances and Disease Registry (ATSDR) reports that four million tons of lead used in gasoline remains in our dust and soil. The Department of Housing and Urban Development (HUD) estimates that three million tons of lead (not lead paint, *lead*) remains on the walls of almost 60 million private housing units—that's three-quarters of all the housing in America. The various bans on the use of lead simply mean we're not adding even more lead pollution to the environment. Unfortunately, there's plenty there already, and lead poisoning is going to be with us for quite a while.

perched on a ladder or sitting on the floor scraping and painting as we rushed to complete renovations before the baby was born. Everyone worried about her falling off the ladder, or breathing in paint fumes. No one knew or thought to question the lead dust and lead fumes we were generating by stripping and scraping layers of paint from our woodwork.

The child exposed to lead in utero is often born prematurely. The risk of delivery before the 37th week of pregnancy if the mother's blood-lead level is 14 μg/dl or higher is almost nine times the risk at levels up to 8 μg/dl. Birth weight, chest circumference, and length/height may all be reduced. Lead's effect on stature has been observed at concentrations as low as 4 μg/dl. Lead poisoning also causes a loss of hearing, with the ability to hear high frequencies affected first.

Babies who are exposed to even low levels of lead in the womb also have been found to have mental and behavioral impairments. Studies in Cincinnati and Boston showed that scores on two key intelligence tests were inversely related to prenatal lead exposure. When six-month-olds were tested, there were significant differences in the scores of low (1.8 μg/dl) and high (14.6 μg/dl) children on the Bayley MDI (Mental Development Index). The Cincinnati study showed a drop of eight points for every 10 μg/dl increase in blood-lead level. The studies indicate that *prenatal* exposure to lead may have an even greater impact than an equal level of exposure in the first few months after birth.

HOW LEAD AFFECTS EARLY CHILDHOOD DEVELOPMENT

A child's blood-lead levels remain relatively constant for the first six months of life, then begin a sharp increase, which continues until the child is 24 months old. The greatest accumulation of lead occurs in the second year of life. Dr. Julian Chisholm of the Kennedy Krieger Institute in Baltimore, one of the pioneers in the field, says the best indicator of how well a child will do on standardized tests given at age 10 will be that child's blood-lead level at 24 months. Dr. Chisholm believes there is a reason.

He explains that during the second year of life, the human brain reorganizes itself. It makes new connections, called synapses, in the nerve pathways. Nerve pathways, along which the brain sends its information, are not unbroken trails. They stop and start, and synapses bridge the gaps. Information is handed over at the synapse, like a relay runner's baton. Lead interferes with building the bridges. The information-baton cannot be passed. Chisholm believes this is the period when the child is most vulnerable to the effects of lead.

Unfortunately, this is also the time when a baby's normal behavior—gumming, teething, and excessive hand-to-mouth activity—makes ingesting lead more likely. Infants crawl. They pick up lead dust from the floor, from their toys, and from pets. Then they put their hands in their mouths, they eat with their hands, they suck their thumbs.

If you ever ran your hand over the outside of a house as a child and happened to taste the white chalk residue, you may recall that the lead compound used in paint tastes sweet, encouraging small children to lick or chew it.

Lead's greatest impact is on the developing child's brain and central nervous system. There have been at least 14 studies, in a number of countries, all measuring lead's impact on the child's intelligence quotient (IQ). There are some inconsistencies in the findings, in part because the negative effect of lead can be offset by what researchers call "confounding factors," but the weight of all the evidence clearly indicates that lead interferes with a child's ability to learn. As you would expect, studies indicate that the more lead the child is exposed to, the more the child's IQ is lowered.

Cultural nourishment during the developmental years can offset the negative effects of both pre- and postnatal lead exposure. It's one of those confounding factors that researchers have to consider in measuring the impact of low-level lead poisoning. Stimulation during these early years—interplay between the parent and child, the availability of toys, reading and talking to the child—directly improves the child's intelligence and later performance in school. I used to tease Andrea that she belonged to the Ben and Jerry School of Child Development because of all the black-and-white shapes she used to decorate Matthew's room. She had read that infants don't recognize colors but are stimulated by black-and-white objects and designs.

It turns out that everything that enriches your child becomes especially important if the child has been exposed to lead. But keep in mind that the best you can do is offset the effects of lead as long as the child remains exposed. The sooner you stop your child's intake of lead, the greater effect cultural enrichment can have.

Lead's attack on intelligence is is just one facet of its impact on the developing child. As noted earlier, it also causes behavioral problems, including irritability and hyperactivity. There may be attention deficit disorders, in which the child is unable to control his or her impulses and is easily distracted. If unrecognized and unmanaged, the behavioral problems often exacerbate the learning problems, leading to negative reinforcement that almost guarantees academic failure.

RELATIONSHIP BETWEEN LEAD AND ACADEMIC PERFORMANCE: THE NEEDLEMAN STUDY

Lead poisoning has a direct effect on a child's success in school. Dr. Herbert Needleman, another pioneer in the field, studied some 12,000 children in Boston, comparing their careers in school with the amount of lead found in the baby teeth they had shed in early grade school. (Since we know that lead is stored in teeth, examining baby teeth is one way to measure early lead exposure.) Dr. Needleman's study shows that a student's success in school is inversely related to the level of lead exposure; the more lead the preschool child absorbed, the worse the child did later in school. Lead levels in teeth that exceeded 20 ppm were linked with a sevenfold risk of becoming a high school dropout. There was a sixfold risk of having a reading disability, vocabulary deficits, problems with attention, and loss of fine motor coordination. Predictably, there was greater absenteeism and lower class ranking. (A recent Danish study has found higher rates of learning disabilities among students with even lower tooth-lead levels.)

Dr. Needleman's study found a downward shift of four to six IQ points. When the individual scores were plotted on a graph, the enormity of the loss became apparent. Not one child achieved superior function, meaning a verbal IQ score of greater than 125. At the other end of the scale, there was a marked increase in the number of kids with severe deficits, meaning a score of less than 80. A four-point downward shift in IQ scores results in a 50 percent increase in the number of retarded children. This lowering of intelligence of an entire generation has significant implications for the future of our society.

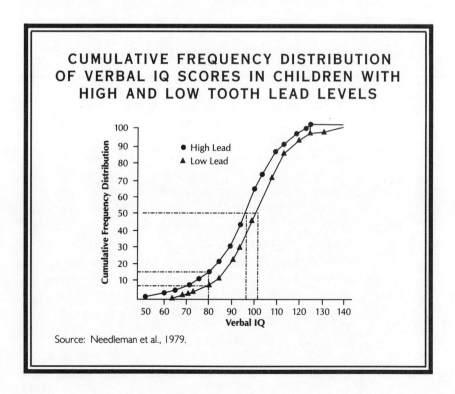

CUMULATIVE FREQUENCY DISTRIBUTION OF VERBAL IQ SCORES IN CHILDREN WITH HIGH AND LOW TOOTH LEAD LEVELS

Source: Needleman et al., 1979.

It must be noted that Needleman's initial study came under intense attack from the lead industry. The industry said that Needleman failed to consider all the confounding factors, including age, poverty, parental neglect (or, conversely, cultural nourishment). Needleman was formally accused of doctoring the results to make lead seem more dangerous. The Needleman study was meticulously investigated by a University of Pittsburgh ethics panel and by the Environmental Protection Agency (EPA). Both cleared him of all charges of scientific misconduct. The charges were then taken to the federal government's Office of Research Integrity. That office also cleared him of any charges of misconduct but criticized his description of the study and recommended that he publish a correction.

Needleman's description of his methodology may have been flawed, but his conclusions were not. The correction, published September 1, 1994, notes that his reporting errors "had no effect on the data analyses performed or the conclusions drawn." Fourteen separate studies have borne out his findings, and a National Academy of Sciences study of low-level lead poisoning concluded that the weight of evidence gathered during the 1980s clearly supported Needleman's conclusions.

LEAD POISONING AND CRIMINALITY

Brace yourself for a new defense on Court TV: lead poisoning. Law professor Deborah Denno of Fordham University in New York City was studying patterns of criminality and discovered a striking connection between lead poisoning and male criminality. Her exhaustive study tracked almost one thousand individuals of both sexes from birth (at the same Philadelphia hospital) until they were twenty-four years old. The size of the study allowed her to test many different theories of crime: "Particularly striking," she wrote*, "among males, lead poisoning, a factor related to the urban environment, was among the strongest predictors of crime, even though numerous biological and psychological factors were also considered." And when Professor Denno tracked the major predictors of criminality across the progression from disciplinary problems in school to juvenile crime to adult crime, lead poisoning was the *only* factor common to all three.

*Fordham Urban Law Journal, Volume XX, Number 3, 1993.

HOW LEAD ATTACKS THE BODY

Other physical ramifications for the young child include anemia and, at higher levels, kidney damage. Lead interferes with the child's ability to produce and use vitamin D, essential for the building of normal teeth and bones, and it inhibits the formation of red blood cells. Children with elevated blood-lead levels may have slowed reaction times, problems with their balance and posture, and may be delayed in the age at which they first sit up, walk, and achieve other developmental mileposts.

Lead accumulates in the human body. The level of toxicity depends on how much lead you—or your child—or both—are exposed to and how long the exposure continues. Lead tricks the body. It bonds to red blood cells in the same way that iron does. It also mimics calcium, and so is taken up and stored in teeth and bones. Almost 95 percent of the body's total accumulated lead is stored in its bones. Bones are the body's calcium warehouse. When calcium levels in the body drop, bones recycle calcium back into the bloodstream for distribution to the liver, brain, and other soft tissue organs. Bones do the same with stored lead. As the blood-lead level goes down, the bone warehouse puts lead back into the bloodstream. Purging the body of lead toxicity can take a long time.

Predictably, iron or calcium deficiencies increase the amount of lead the body absorbs. Iron deficiency has long been recognized as a major factor in the high level of lead absorption among the children of poor, inner-city families. Sickle cell anemia is another complicating factor in the inner city. Sickle cell causes a deficiency in zinc, which increases both the absorption and toxicity risk of lead. Deficiencies in protein and phosphorus also increase the rate of lead retention.

Your child's ability to absorb ingested lead can be limited by making sure she or he gets enough iron and calcium. A diet high in iron and calcium (especially iron) can play a critical role in limiting low-level lead poisoning.

The relationship between cause and effect—how much ingested lead results in how high a blood-lead level—is affected by a number of variables. The body absorbs different forms of lead at different rates. Different parts of the body absorb lead at different rates. And, as we've seen, nutrition affects absorption rates. However, the most important variable is age, and there are two factors working against kids.

Children retain a far greater percentage of the lead they're exposed to than do adults. This starts before birth and continues up to age seven, when the retention rate falls off quickly. Older children and adults can be exposed to four times as much lead as a young child before they will reach the same blood-lead level. This high rate of lead retention comes at the same time the child is developing, both mentally and physically. As a result, even low levels of lead have a greater effect. Whereas lead affects young children at blood levels as low as 10 μg/dl, the first measurable effects on adults occur at about 30 μg/dl.

The Food and Drug Administration (FDA) has put together a chart that relates daily lead ingestion to lead poisoning in children and adults (see table). The figures represent *total* intake, not just intake from food or water or some other source; lead poisoning is cumulative. These are estimates of the amount of lead that will push the lead concentration in blood to the CDC action levels. There's a separate line for pregnant women because the fetus shares the mother's blood-lead level and so the mother's blood-lead level must not exceed 10 μg/dl. You want to stay as far below these intake levels as possible.

The most dangerous form of lead pollution is airborne lead. This includes lead-paint dust and lead vapors created by burning off old paint, burning lead-painted wood, soldering and melting lead for use in various hobbies. It also includes out-of-the-home industrial sources. Your lungs absorb between 30 and 50 percent of the lead you breathe in. Children's lungs absorb at the same rate as adults, but kids have a higher metabolic rate. That means they breathe in more air, relative to

DAILY LEVELS OF LEAD INGESTION RESULTING IN LEAD POISONING

POPULATION	LEAD INGESTED (μG/DAY)	CONVERSION FACTOR*	BLOOD-LEAD LEVEL (μG/DL)
Children ages 0–7	60	0.16	10
Pregnant women	250	0.04	10
Adults	750	0.04	30

*The conversion factor represents the relative rate at which lead is absorbed by the body. As a quick rule of thumb, every 6 μg of lead that a child ingests will raise his or her blood-lead level by 1 μg/dl.

their body size and weight, than adults. It's estimated that children's lungs absorb two to three times as much lead as adults.

Burning material contaminated with lead is extremely hazardous. During the Depression, junkyards recycling lead gave discarded battery casings to poor people to be used as fuel. The practice led to an outbreak of lead poisoning in Baltimore that came to be called the "Depression Disease." The Depression ended, but poverty did not, and lead poisoning from this source has been reported into the 1980s. Burning colored newsprint or wood coated with lead paint can also release lead into the air.

The high rate at which airborne lead enters the body explains why leaded gasoline was such a hazard. As cars burned the gas, the entire lead content passed out through the exhaust and into the atmosphere. Air became one of the primary paths by which lead entered people's bodies. After the EPA ordered the phasing out of leaded gasoline in 1976, researchers charting blood-lead levels found a startlingly close correlation between the reduction in use of leaded gasoline and a decline in the levels of lead in blood.

Animal research shows that the smaller the particles of lead, the more easily they'll be absorbed. In experiments with rats, when the size of the ingested lead dropped from 150 to 8 microns—a micron is one millionth of a meter—the rate of absorption increased 500 percent. This explains why lead-paint dust that you can't see may be even more dangerous than lead-paint chips. While both the particle size and the chemical form of the lead in dust affect the rate at which it's absorbed, the EPA estimates that for every 1,000 ppm increase in the amount of lead in dust, there is a 3 to 7 μg/dl rise in the level of lead in the blood.

TAKE THE INITIATIVE IN PROTECTING YOUR CHILD

The decision of the CDC to set 10 μg/dl as the "threshold of concern" was based on practicality. The ability to measure at lower levels is imprecise. The research is so new that scientists haven't identified and evaluated ways to deal with lead at these low levels. And the CDC admits we would be overwhelmed by the sheer numbers of affected children if the threshold were lowered farther. The government is practicing preventive triage. It's focusing attention and resources first on those with the most serious problems. Even so, the CDC sees 10 μg/dl as a start, not a finish. Prevention activities, it says, should work to reduce children's blood-lead levels *at least* to below 10 μg/dl.

The government is dealing with almost two million kids; you and I are dealing only with our own. The government has a 20-year society-wide plan to eliminate lead poisoning; you and I can't wait. Unlike Uncle Sam, we have the opportunity to remove every possible source of lead exposure and to get our children's blood-lead levels as low as possible . . . right now.

2

TESTING AND TREATMENT

*Most lead poisoned children do not
show symptoms that are easily
diagnosed. If you wait until your child
has overt symptoms, it is too late—the
damage is probably already done.*

—*Alliance to End Childhood
Lead Poisoning*

OUR FIRST REACTION to Matthew's test results was total shock, followed by panic, fear, and guilt. The CDC had just lowered the "threshold of concern" to 10 µg/dl, and Matthew's level was double that. What had we done? What was happening to our baby? Not a year earlier, we'd mortgaged ourselves to the hilt to secure a nice home and neighborhood in which to raise a child. Now, in a single phone call, we learned that our sanctuary had a curse on it. Our house became the enemy: Every minute Matthew spent in it, he was being slowly and surely poisoned.

Our first concern was Matthew. Our pediatrician provided us with a basic plan of action and some reassurance. We had caught the problem relatively early, before much damage had been done. Still, we can't escape the knowledge that Matthew must have lost something to his lead exposure. He was in the low 20s at 18 months, well above the "maybe, maybe not" level, and we are left to always wonder. Fortunately, Matthew is turning out to be a bright, cheerful, and well-behaved little boy. That makes it easier to leave behind the "If only we'd known" recriminations, and concentrate instead on the "Thank goodness we caught it as quickly as we did" side of things. We still wish we'd caught it sooner.

The CDC advocates universal screening—the routine blood-lead testing of every young child. The argument is simple: Lead poisoning, if diagnosed, can be reversed. It can be treated. The earlier lead poisoning is diagnosed, the less impact it will have. Universal screening could eradicate lead poisoning.

Critics say this would be too expensive. But like most aspects of preventive medicine, the cost of detecting and preventing lead poisoning is far less than the price we are now paying to deal with the consequences of the disease.

If all children were screened, a data base could be established, providing a statistical base for more intensive scientific research. It would also help educators and social workers, since lead poisoning is associated with such problems as learning disabilities and behavioral disorders, which they encounter on a regular basis.

A national data base would also help determine public policy by giving definitive evidence of how large a problem lead poisoning is and how we could best allocate limited public resources to target intervention for the greatest number of children at high risk.

While the government debates the issue, the physical and mental health of the next generation is at great risk. It is important for parents of young children and for pregnant women to take the initiative in testing their offspring for lead poisoning.

Such testing of individual children could have a positive snowball effect on the health of other children. Diagnosing one case of lead poisoning is often a catalyst for identifying and testing siblings or playmates who may have been exposed to the same contamination. And removing the source of one child's lead poisoning protects the rest of the children in that environment, whether it's a home or a day-care center or even an entire community.

Testing is the *only* way to detect lead poisoning in time to prevent or limit permanent damage. Parents usually report there were no symptoms, no one suspected . . . until a serendipitous test revealed lead lurking in the child's blood.

If the test comes back below 10 μg/dl—*and most will*—you can feel assured your child is not being poisoned by lead.

An elevated level, however, is not an irreversible diagnosis. The threat of lead poisoning is out in the open, and you can take steps to halt low-level lead poisoning. Even acute lead poisoning can be treated. All levels can be brought down. The sooner you find out you have the problem and start preventive action, the better.

In certain cases, it is advisable to test for lead poisoning even before a child is conceived. If a woman planning to become pregnant has been exposed to lead, either by paint in the home or through an occupation or hobby, she should be tested as soon as possible.

WHEN DO I TEST MY CHILD?

There is seldom a reason to test a child younger than six months. The CDC recommends starting testing at six months for children at high risk (see box), and at 12 to 15 months for children at lower risk.

Continue annual testing at least through age three. Testing should continue or be resumed past age three if the child is exposed to lead (see box), or if the child is lead poisoned, in which case your health care-provider should schedule frequent testing. Blood-lead levels seem to peak (if the exposure remains constant) at 24 months.

THE CHILDREN AT GREATEST RISK

According to the CDC, children from the ages of six to 72 months who fall into one or more of the following groups run the highest risk of being lead poisoned:
—Living in or paying frequent visits to deteriorated housing built before 1960.
—Living in or paying frequent visits to housing built before 1960 where there is recent, ongoing, or planned renovation or remodeling.
—Having siblings, housemates, or playmates known to have lead poisoning.
—Having parents or other household members who participate in a lead-related occupation or hobby.
—Living near active lead smelters, battery recycling plants, or other industries likely to release lead into the atmosphere.

Some experts say there is no need to test beyond the age of three if earlier tests have shown no exposure to lead. Others, arguing that children start nursery school or other out-of-home activities at about this age and could then be exposed to new sources of lead, recommend testing through age six.

The CDC screening schedule is conservative, recognizing limited resources while establishing national priorities. As a parent, your priority is your child's well-being, so if there is any reason to suspect your child could have been exposed to lead, have the test performed at an earlier age, or more frequently, or until your child is older than six. Follow your own instincts, along with your pediatrician's advice.

We wish we had had our son tested sooner. Matthew's first test, at 16 months, revealed a blood-lead level of 21 μg/dl. A confirmatory test, taken six weeks after the first one, showed that his lead level had increased, but only slightly, up to 23 μg/dl. By then, we had started to completely inventory potential lead sources in our home, and we had taken initial remedial steps, including replacing tap water with bottled water for anything he would eat or drink. (Subsequent chapters of this book will show you how to lead-proof your house and lessen your child's exposure to lead outside the home.) Our pediatrician advised against taking any drastic action— like moving out of our house—until we'd had a chance to see what effect our initial steps might have. When Matthew went back for his third test three months later, his blood-lead level was down to the magic 10 μg/dl. It can happen that quickly!

WHERE CAN I GET MY CHILD TESTED?

Lead testing should be a part of regular child well-care, but you should be prepared to ask your pediatrician. Don't rely on the doctor to broach the subject. Awareness of both the dangers and prevalence of low-level lead poisoning is still new, but any pediatrician or pediatric nurse should be able to offer blood-lead testing.

Ask if an area hospital or clinic runs a lead poisoning program. Montefiore Hospital in New York City charges $8 for a blood-lead test, including taking the blood sample. This is significantly less than what private labs generally charge. (The lab work on Matthew's blood cost $55 when his doctor drew the blood sample. There would have been an additional $10 charge if the lab had drawn the blood sample.)

In addition to saving money at a lead clinic, you will generally get the results more quickly. Montefiore reports in one to two days; many parents wait one to two weeks for reports from private labs.

In Massachusetts, which mandates lead screening, most blood samples are sent to a state laboratory for analysis. The cost is $20. Results below 20 µg/dl are mailed back, but for any sample testing over 20 µg/dl, notification is given by phone within 24 hours.

Most health-care plans will pay for lead screening, but private medical insurance will pay for lead testing only if the policy includes a provision for child well-care. An Alliance to End Childhood Lead Poisoning study of health insurance coverage found that only health maintenance organizations (HMOs), which cover approximately 20 percent of all children, consistently cover lead screening. Children in Head Start, WIC (Women, Infants, and Children), and some other public assistance programs may get free screening as part of their program. Many localities offer free lead screening clinics annually or even semi-annually. Check with your local health department.

HOW IS THE BLOOD TESTED?

There are a number of different tests for lead poisoning, of varying degree of accuracy and difficulty. One of the major goals of researchers in this area is to come up with a test that is accurate at low levels, easy to administer, and inexpensive.

The EP or FEP (for free erythrocyte protoporphyrin) test measures a chemical that changes when exposed to lead. This test is no longer recommended as a screen for lead poisoning. That's because it's not sensitive enough to identify lead levels below 25 µg/dl. Moreover, a high EP reading is not a definitive test for lead poisoning because several other health conditions can cause an elevated EP reading, including iron deficiency. In fact, EP tests are used to screen for iron deficiencies by many nutritional programs (the WIC Program, for instance). If these tests show lead poisoning, they indicate significant exposure, but remember that an EP test that comes up lead-free is meaningless.

Blood-lead measurement is now the accepted means of screening for lead poisoning because the level of lead in the blood is an accurate indicator of recent exposure to lead. It is less accurate in determining either past or cumulative exposure, since half of the lead that enters your blood today will be gone (some excreted, the rest deposited in bones) about a month from now.

The problem with blood testing is getting the blood. There are two ways to get a sample, and there are drawbacks to both. The easiest way is the classic finger prick. A nurse or doctor pricks the child's finger and collects drops of blood. (Puncturing the skin of an infant under one year of age for the collection of a blood sample is usually done in the heel, not the finger.)

The disadvantage of the finger-prick test is that the blood can easily be contaminated with lead dust that may be on the child's finger, resulting in a false-high reading. But because it is easier and less expensive to do, finger-prick testing is quite common. However, while finger-prick tests are helpful for screening, the CDC says that any finger-prick sample that results in an elevated blood-lead level must be followed up with the more accurate venous blood test.

Medical interventions are *always* based on the results of venous blood-lead levels. The needle-in-the-vein (venous or venipuncture) blood sample is much less susceptible to the contamination that can lead to false-high readings but is more demanding. Since it is difficult to get a needle into the tiny veins of an infant or small child, some pediatricians in larger communities may refer you to a laboratory to have the venous blood sample drawn.

Today's equipment and techniques can successfully measure levels of lead as low as 2 to 5 μg/dl, but the reading could be several μg/dl above or below the actual level of lead in the blood. Since the margin

THE XRF LEAD TEST

Blood screening gives a snapshot of a child's lead exposure. It tells you what is happening right now. A different kind of test, X-ray flourescence (XRF), measures the level of lead in bones.

Since bones store lead, XRF testing measures cumulative, or historic, lead exposure. Andrew C. Todd, Ph.D., assistant professor of community medicine at New York's Mt. Sinai Hospital, says XRF testing is a complement, not a replacement, for blood-lead testing. XRF testing is still very new, and Professor Todd hopes to study the relationship of bone-lead levels to attention disorders and hyperactivity. *Another area needing study is what happens to bone levels after chelation treatment.*

CDC LEAD POISONING CLASSIFICATION

CLASS	BLOOD-LEAD LEVEL (μG/DL)
I	Under 10
IIA	10–14
IIB	15–19
III	20–44
IV	45–69
V	Over 69

of error tends to be consistent within a given laboratory, it's best to stick with one lab if you're tracing the history of a particular child's lead levels.

All of Matthew's blood samples were taken from the vein. The early ones were drawn in the doctor's office, but when it came time for his three-year test, his doctor asked my wife, Andrea, to take Matthew directly to the lab to have the blood sample drawn. Andrea asked why; the doctor explained that she didn't want him to associate her with pain and fear! Kids don't like needles any more than you do. Pediatricians suggest that you prepare yourself and your child for the procedure. The needle will hurt and your child will cry, but it will be over very quickly, and your little one will get to wear a Band-Aid! The healing powers of a Sesame Street or Ninja Turtle adhesive bandage are not to be underestimated!

There is no consensus on what constitutes lead poisoning. The 10 μg/dl level, set by the CDC in October 1991 as the "threshold of concern," is now used by most as the start point for lead poisoning. However, Dr. Sue Binder, chief of the CDC's Lead Poisoning Branch, says the CDC does not refer to cases below 15 μg/dl as being "poisoned." Some literature, including government fact sheets, refer to blood-lead levels below 10 μg/dl as "normal." Levels below 10 μg/dl may be common today, but they are hardly normal; there is no "normal" level of lead in the human body.

The CDC has established six classes of lead poisoning based on blood-lead levels (see chart). Most children's results should come back below 10 μg/dl. Statistically, ATSDR estimates that more than 90 per-

DO THE EASY THINGS FIRST

Careful housekeeping and good nutrition are a parent's first lines of defense against lead poisoning. One reduces exposure; the other limits uptake. Your child's exposure to ingested lead can be lowered by doing the following:

- Wash your hands before preparing the child's food.
- Wash the child's hands before serving the food.
- Wash bottle nipples and pacifiers frequently, especially if they fall on the floor.
- Wash the child's toys frequently.
- Stomp your feet before coming in the house to clean your shoes of outside soil that may carry lead from exterior house paint.
- Damp-mop frequently along baseboards, around door frames, under windowsills and, if you have them, iron radiators.
- Wash windowsills and wells frequently. (The well is the depression behind the sill where the window fits when it's closed.) Move the crib away from the window. Children chew windowsills, and window wells collect lead paint dust.
- Always damp-mop before vacuuming. Home vacuum cleaners don't trap lead dust; they blow it into the air.

When washing, use a product such as LEDIZOLV (available in hardware stores), which is formulated to bind and remove lead particles. If you can't find this, then use a *phosphate* detergent. Read labels to find a high-phosphate detergent. Dish-washing detergents are often high-

cent of the children in America *will not* test above the 10 μg/dl threshold.

Lower levels of lead poisoning usually require a systematic approach to reduction and prevention, starting with examining nutritional practices and housekeeping measures (see box). There are many potential lead sources, but begin by looking for lead paint, either in chip or dust form. Paint is almost always a prime source of lead poisoning. But don't stop there. Your child is probably being exposed to lead from a combination of sources.

phosphate. So is TSP (Tri-Sodium Phosphate), sold in hardware stores. Mix two teaspoons of phosphate detergent in each gallon of warm water. Laundry detergents generally do not contain phosphates and will not pick up dust particles of lead.

Your child's ability to absorb ingested lead can be limited by making sure she or he gets enough iron and calcium. A diet high in iron and calcium (especially iron) can play a critical role in limiting low-level lead poisoning.

Although the CDC recommends feeding your toddler liver, fortified cereal, cooked legumes, and spinach for iron and milk, yogurt, cheese, and cooked greens for calcium, most of this is not likely to go down well with the typical two-year-old. Your doctor can recommend an iron supplement to help bring the lead level down. Raisin bran cereal, Ovaltine chocolate drink, peanut butter, apples, chicken and turkey, baked potatoes, hot chocolate, ice milk, and pudding all are rich sources of iron or calcium and are foods a finicky youngster might eat.

Vitamin C also helps limit lead absorption. Sweet potatoes, cantaloupe, and strawberries were hits with our son, Matthew.

You should avoid fried and fatty foods, including french fries, fried chicken, and potato chips, since fats helps the body retain lead.

Make sure your child eats often enough; simply keeping the tummy full helps retard lead absorption.

Finally, unless you have had a lead test done on the *cold* water coming from your kitchen faucet, use bottled water for formula and food preparation for your child (see chapter 6). Never use hot water from the tap for either formula or food for your infant or toddler.

Complete medical evaluations are necessary for any child with a blood-lead level of 20 µg/dl or above, although medical treatment generally isn't called for until blood-lead levels hit 45 µg/dl or more. At these levels, immediate action must be taken to reduce the child's exposure to lead. Most lead poisoning happens at home and may come from as simple a source as a lead-glazed pitcher used to store a baby's juice. When reducing the exposure requires extensive work such as the removal of old leaded paint from a house or apartment, it is important that the child (and all young children and pregnant women) be relocated until the work is done, since lead-paint dust is extremely hazard-ous and will worsen the child's condition.

WHAT THE RESULTS MEAN AND WHAT YOU SHOULD DO

CLASS I (under 10 μg/dl)

What it means: If your child tests 9 μg/dl or under, you are at or about the national average, and your child is not considered to be lead poi-soned. No medical attention is needed, and your child should not be affected by this level of lead exposure.

What to do: Continue good nutrition and housekeeping practices, at the same time remaining on guard against unnecessary lead expo-sure, both in and out of your home.

Retesting: If your child is at low risk, retest at 12 and 24 months of age. Testing at 24 months is most important, for this is when blood-lead levels peak. If your child is at *high risk* (see box, p. 17) and you are not able to change whatever conditions pose the threat of lead poisoning, your child should be retested every six months, at least until the age of three. If two consecutive tests come back under 10 μg/dl or three come back under 15 μg/dl, testing can be cut back to once a year.

CLASS IIA (10–14 μg/dl)

What it means: Your child is in a lead poisoning border zone. The accuracy of lab tests are such that the true lead level could still be under 10 μg/dl. There is no need for medical intervention. Adverse effects on learning and behavior at these levels are subtle and may not be measur-able in the individual child.

What to do: Lead poisoning at this level is likely to be an accumula-tion of many small inputs. As with Class I, you want to continue good nutrition and housekeeping practices. Be aggressive about looking for ways to reduce lead exposure. Test your water. Your goal is to keep these levels from increasing, while trying to bring them below 10 μg/dl.

Retesting: Because this is a border zone, testing needs to be done more frequently. Whether *low risk* or *high risk,* your child should be retested every three to four months until two consecutive tests come back under 10 μg/dl or three come back under 15 μg/dl. Then testing can be cut back to once a year.

CLASS IIB (15–19 μg/dl)

What it means: The effects of lead poisoning at this level, while still subtle, are now noticeable if exposure is prolonged. Children at this level are at risk for decreases in intelligence of up to several IQ points. There may be both behavioral and developmental delays. There is still no known medical intervention that is effective at these levels, but your doctor should test for iron deficiency.

What to do: Follow the methods described for Classes I and IIA to reduce your child's exposure to lead. You need to take a full inventory of potential sources of lead exposure and move quickly to either remove them or remove your child from them. Switch immediately to bottled water for formula and other uses until testing shows your water to be free of lead.

Retesting: If these are the results of a finger-prick test, they should be confirmed by a venous test *within one month.* All subsequent tests should be on blood drawn from the vein. Your child should be retested every three to four months until three consecutive tests come back under 15 μg/dl or two come back under 10 μg/dl, when testing can be cut back to once a year.

COMMON SYMPTOMS OF LEAD POISONING

As the level of lead toxicity increases, the child will develop one or more of the following symptoms:

- Headaches
- Cramps
- Constipation
- Poor appetite
- Crankiness
- Clumsiness

- Stomachaches
- Vomiting
- Anorexia
- Sleep disorders
- Fatigue and lethargy
- No interest in play

Many of these symptoms are the same as for a cold, the flu, or other childhood maladies. *A blood-lead test is the only way to diagnose lead poisoning.*

CLASS III (20–44 μg/dl)

What it means: Your child needs a full medical evaluation, including a detailed behavioral and developmental history. Class III covers a wide range of lead poisoning and is the transition stage between low-level and acute toxicity. The need for medical attention becomes more urgent at the upper levels of blood-lead poisoning or if there are visible symptoms (see box). Your child's abdomen may be x-rayed to see if a swallowed object (lead shot, curtain weight, fishing sinker, or even paint chips) is contributing to the elevated blood-lead levels. A single swallowed lead object has been known to cause low- to moderate-level lead poisoning. Hearing should be tested.

Your doctor should conduct a full physical examination, as well as a hearing test and a test for iron deficiency. You will need to discuss with the doctor your child's language development and any reading or other learning disabilities your child might have. If your child is in day care or preschool, talk to the caregiver or teacher in order to get their observations and to alert them to potential problems.

What to do: Conduct a full environmental survey. This means aggressively looking for every possible source of lead exposure, not just in your home but wherever your child spends time. In many localities, a lead level this high triggers intervention by local health officials who will help you determine the lead source. If they don't come automatically, call them. If they don't have an expert who can help, they should be able to direct you to one. If they can't help at all, call the state lead contact number listed in appendix D. You must immediately remove or reduce lead sources. At the upper end of this classification, it may be necessary to remove the child from the lead environment until the source of lead can be removed or encapsulated. Switch immediately to bottled water for formula and other uses until testing shows your water to be free of lead. If the source of lead is found to be in a public place, such as lead paint in a playground or day-care center or apartment-house hallway, it's important that local health officials be notified quickly so that the risk to all children, including your own, can be eliminated. Other children under the age of seven who share the same exposure as the lead-poisoned child should have their blood-lead levels tested.

Treatment with chelation (pronounced key-lay-tion) — the use of certain drugs called chelating agents to flush lead out of the system — is generally not called for at the low end of Class III. Some clinics will use Cuprimine as a chelating agent when blood-lead levels reach the upper range of the classification.

Retesting: If these are the results of a finger-prick test, they should be confirmed by a venous test *immediately.* All subsequent tests should be on blood drawn from the vein. Your child should be retested every three to four months until three consecutive tests come back under 15 μg/dl or two come back under 10 μg/dl, when testing can be cut back to once a year.

CLASS IV (45–69 μg/dl)

What it means: Your child requires a full medical evaluation, including a detailed behavioral and developmental history. There may be physical symptoms of lead poisoning (see box, p. 25). Unless your health-care provider has a lot of experience with this problem, ask to be referred to a clinic specializing in managing serious lead poisoning cases.

What to do: Seek help from public-health lead-poisoning specialists in identifying and eliminating sources of lead contamination. Your child's exposure to lead should be stopped immediately. If possible, send your child to live with a relative or friend *in a known lead-free environment* until the source(s) of lead has been eliminated. Many hospitals and clinics now provide temporary lead-free housing for you and your child to live in while the sources of lead are being eliminated from your home. Detoxicated children must never be returned to a lead-contaminated environment.

Removing the child from the source of lead should start to bring levels down, but chelation treatment may still be called for. Doctors may run a test (an Edetate Disodium Calcium Provocative Chelation Test) to determine whether chelation would be effective. A dose of the chelating agent is administered, and then the amount of lead excreted over an eight-hour period is measured. While chelation is very effective with lead levels over 70 μg/dl, studies with the Provocative Chelation Test show that chelation would be effective with 76 percent of all children having levels of 35 to 44 μg/dl and only 35 percent of the children having levels of 25 to 34 μg/dl.

Even with oral chelating agents, children are normally hospitalized until their blood-lead level is brought below 45 μg/dl.

Other children under the age of seven who share the same exposure as the lead-poisoned child should have their blood-lead levels tested.

Retesting: If these are the results of a finger-prick test, they should be confirmed by a venous test *immediately.* All subsequent tests should be on blood drawn from the vein. Retesting will be frequent until blood-lead levels are brought down to at least Class III levels. At that point, your child should be retested every three to four months until three consecutive tests come back under 15 µg/dl or two come back under 10 µg/dl, when testing can be cut back to once a year.

CLASS V (over 69 µg/dl)

What it means: This is a medical emergency. Your child is critically ill, probably showing distinct physical symptoms of lead poisoning (see box). Your child needs immediate attention from people experienced in treating children with lead poisoning.

Brain damage (acute lead encephalopathy) has been noted at levels as low as 70 µg/dl and is almost certain as levels approach 100 µg/dl. Even with prompt treatment, lead poisoning at these elevated levels will cause severe and permanent brain damage in 70 to 80 percent of affected children.

What to do: Immediately remove your child from the lead exposure. Get your child to a clinic or hospital experienced in chelation

---

SYMPTOMS OF ACUTE LEAD POISONING

At blood levels of 70 µg/dl and up in children, some or all of the following symptoms may be present:

- Bizarre behavior
- Apathy
- Vomiting
- Loss of muscular coordination
- Loss of recently acquired skills

If the brain has been affected (acute lead encephalopathy), it may also cause:

- Altered state of consciousness
- Seizures
- Coma

Untreated, acute lead poisoning can lead to death.

therapy. Chelation therapy should begin immediately, without waiting for any confirmatory retesting. Work quickly with professionals to identify and eliminate the source of lead poisoning. Your child must not be returned to the source of lead poisoning.

Everyone, especially other children but also adults (including you), who is exposed to the same lead source or environment should be tested for lead poisoning. At the very least, this would include everyone who shares your home. Be sure to test any children who regularly visit or play in your home, and if you live in an apartment building or housing complex with similar units, testing should be extensive. Local public health officials should be notified automatically by the doctor or lab, but if they aren't, call them.

Retesting: A venous test should be done immediately. Venous retesting will be frequent until blood-lead levels are brought down to at least the lower range of Class III levels (20–44 µg/dl). At that point, your child should be retested every three to four months until three consecutive tests come back under 15 µg/dl or two come back under 10 µg/dl, when testing can be cut back to once a year.

Treatment for acute lead poisoning will require a team of professionals, which may include specialists in critical care, toxicology, neurology, and neurosurgery.

CHELATION THERAPY

Chelation therapy takes time and money. At the Kennedy Krieger Institute in Baltimore, chelation treatment requires 28 days in the hospital. Blood-lead levels ride a roller coaster during chelation treatment. Chelation is done in cycles. At the end of each cycle, the blood-lead level usually drops below 25 µg/dl. As the body seeks equilibrium, lead stored in the bones is released, and the blood-lead level goes back up. Chelation may have to be repeated several times. The CDC recommends checking blood-lead levels 7 to 21 days after chelation to see if retreatment is needed.

The CDC lists four chelating agents used to treat lead poisoning. Three are FDA approved; one is not.

Cuprimine, with the generic name D-penicillamine, is not FDA approved for chelating lead (although it is approved for other uses), but it is used by some clinics to remove lead from children with blood levels under 45 µg/dl. It enhances the excretion of lead in urine and has the advantage of being an oral medication. It's available as tablets or capsules; capsules can be opened and suspended in a liquid. Dosage is increased gradually to minimize side effects. It can be given over a long period of time. It may be prescribed for administration at home, but the CDC warns doctors not to do this if there is continuing exposure to lead, or if the doctor believes the dosage regimen cannot be carefully followed.

Cuprimine requires careful monitoring since up to 33 percent of patients given the drug have side effects similar to those for penicillin. Doctors are most concerned about the possibility of kidney damage. *Cuprimine cannot be given to anyone with a known penicillin allergy.*

BAL in Oil, with the generic name Dimercaprol, is one of the traditional chelating agents for lead. BAL is available only in peanut oil and is given through intramuscular injection. It increases both fecal and urinary excretion of lead and can be used even if the kidneys have been damaged. BAL is usually administered every four hours, occasionally every eight hours. Between 30 and 50 percent of patients who are given BAL will experience side effects; most are minor and quickly subside. BAL is most often used in cases where blood-lead levels exceed 70 µg/dl, and it may be used in combination with Calcium Disodium Versenate (see below).

There are risks in administering BAL to patients with certain glucose deficiencies, and an iron deficiency cannot be medicated during BAL chelation treatment. *BAL should not be used to treat children allergic to peanuts or peanut products.*

Calcium Disodium Versenate (CaNa$_2$EDTA), with the generic name Edetate disodium calcium, is the other traditional chelating agent. Usually referred to as EDTA, the drug is administered intravenously and increases urinary lead excretion by a factor of anywhere from 20 to 50. It is normally given in a continuous infusion, although it can be given in two intravenous doses per day. EDTA can be given as an intramuscular shot, but the injection is very painful. It cannot be given orally, for it has been shown to increase the absorption of lead from the gastrointestinal tract.

Prolonged use of EDTA is toxic to the kidneys. Treatment is kept to no more than five days, with a two- to five-day break before resumption. In cases with high blood-lead levels (70 µg/dl or more), EDTA used by itself can aggravate the symptoms of lead poisoning, so BAL is usually administered first.

Succimer (pronounced sucks-i-mer), the generic name for the product Chemet, is the newest chelating agent. In January 1991, the FDA approved its use in the treatment of blood-lead levels greater than 45

THE RESEARCH GOES ON . . .

Doctors are learning more about lead poisoning every day. Scientists around the world are studying not only what lead does but how it does it and how that process might be reversed. Some of the more promising recent findings hold out the possibilities of:

■ *A way to stop seizures:* A study at the State University of New York at Binghampton found that a drug used to treat angina, hypertension, and other heart conditions may prevent seizures caused by acute lead poisoning. Researchers found that a medicine, nimodipine, used to treat coronary conditions by preventing the flow of calcium to muscle cells, blocked lead seizures. Now they're trying to figure out how it works.

■ *A way to combat the urge to eat lead:* The same study found that nimodipine destroyed the urge to eat lead. The study was conducted with animals raised to eat lead. When they were given the drug, they stopped eating lead. Scientists think the drug may eventually be used to treat those children who have developed a craving for the "sweet" taste of lead paint.

■ *A better way to teach lead-poisoned children:* Research on learning contracted by the EPA has shown that lead-poisoned animals need more stimulation to learn a specific task than normal animals do. However, once they learned the task, they performed it as well and as long as the control group. The implication is that, given more intellectual stimulation, lead-poisoned children can be brought up to par with their peers.

■ *A way to reverse the damage to brain cells:* Research at the University of Iowa showed that chelators reverse lead's damage to young brain cells. Chelating agents or chelators are drugs used to remove high levels of lead from the body. Experimenting with frogs, the Iowa team found that neurons—brain cells—exposed to lead grew to only 20 percent of their normal size. The chelators reversed this process. Researchers now want to learn why, and at what point in the brain's development the damage can be reversed.

■ *Better ways to screen for lead exposure:* Researchers at New York University have identified five antibodies in the blood that seem to increase in proportion to exposure to lead. The antibodies appear in the blood shortly after exposure and may provide a more accurate means of determining cumulative exposure to lead.

■ *A way to discover lead biomarkers that would permit simpler lead*

> *screening:* Scientists at the University of Maryland at Baltimore are studying changes in calcium-binding proteins, measurable in blood, and lead-binding proteins, measurable in urine. A blood biomarker would allow health-care providers to once again collect blood samples with a simple finger prick, since the potential for contamination would be removed. A urine biomarker would eliminate the need for any invasive sampling. In the meantime, the CDC is working with the private sector to develop a cheaper and easier-to-use method for measuring lead in blood and expects positive results in a couple of years.

μg/dl. Succimer has created much excitement because it can be administered orally and increases urinary excretion of lead by the same high factor as Calcium Disodium Versenate. An added benefit is that it does not remove other (beneficial) metals from the body. Succimer is administered every eight hours for a 19-day period. A two-week lapse is recommended before Succimer treatment is resumed.

The problem with Succimer is that it's very new, and clinicians do not have a great deal of experience with it. Most of the experience to date has been with blood levels of 45 to 69 μg/dl. There has been very limited experience using Succimer at levels over 69 μg/dl. There appear to be few side effects, but this too needs additional monitoring. The Kennedy Krieger Institute is currently testing Succimer on some 300 children under a $5.8-million federal contract.

A child who has undergone chelation treatment needs frequent checkups, including blood-lead testing, for at least one year and often longer. The child must not be reexposed to a lead-contaminated environment. Clinic after clinic report chilling cases where children went through four weeks of hospitalization and chelation, only to return to a lead-laden home. Some were back in the hospital within weeks, forced to start the chelation cycle all over again.

While chelation lowers the level of lead in the body and prevents further damage and loss, it does not reverse what damage has already occurred.

PUBLIC SCREENING PROGRAMS

As awareness of lead poisoning grows, public health programs are becoming proactive. New York State requires well-care screening at one and two years of age, and also requires proof of lead screening within three months of enrollment in a child-care facility, nursery, or pre-school. New York recorded 33,000 children with elevated lead levels in 1992 and expects that number to double once the screening law fully takes effect.

Seven other states, including California, also have some form of lead screening laws on the books. When a child's blood-lead level is 20 μg/dl or greater, Massachusetts sends a licensed inspector to the child's home. Every painted surface, inside and out, is tested for lead. If no lead paint is found, the inspector moves on to water, dust, soil, and any other possible source of poisoning. In Massachusetts, lead paint must be abated *by a licensed contractor.*

New York and Maryland also require local health departments to investigate sources of contamination and recommend ways to reduce the exposure. New York City requires owners of pre-1960 buildings to address lead problems in any building in which a child under the age of six resides. If the landlord doesn't do the work, the city contracts the work and then bills the owner of the building.

Your first and often best source of local lead poisoning information should be your state or local health department. Appendix D is a state-by-state list of official lead information resources. A rapidly improving source of information is the EPA's Lead Hotline, available toll-free at 1-800-LEAD-FYI.

Chelation treatment for lead poisoning is a painful and costly ordeal that no child and no family should have to go through. Lead poisoning is entirely preventable. Early testing can alert you to the presence of lead. The rest of this book will tell you how to eliminate this silent hazard.

3

PAINT

We were much puzzled as to the source of the lead, until he was found with his mouth covered with white lead paint which he had bitten from the railings of his crib.

—Mortality report of 5-year-old child killed by lead poisoning, 1914

SANDRA ROSEBERRY'S three-story white clapboard farmhouse, nestled in the foothills of New Hampshire's White Mountains, looked like the setting of a Norman Rockwell painting. A big wraparound porch caught the fragrance of lilacs and offered protection from spring showers and summer sun. It appeared to be the perfect place to raise children.

Amanda Roseberry was barely 18 months old when her parents bought the house. The porch became her nursery. With gates at either end, she could toddle, and later run, from outside the living room past the dining room to just outside the kitchen, always within her mother's sight—the safest place in the world.

The child was always getting white chalky stuff on her hands while playing on the porch, sometimes from grasping the turned-wood spindles of the period railing, sometimes from just brushing against the clapboard siding. The white stuff got on everything: her clothes, her dolls, her pacifier, her thumb. As a toddler, she'd often have juice and crackers or some other snack out on the porch.

When Amanda was three and a half, nurses at her health clinic asked Sandra Roseberry if Amanda could be tested for lead as part of a random statewide sampling program. Sandra said yes and thought nothing more of it—until the call came two weeks later. Amanda's blood-lead level was past 40 µg/dl.

"Poisoned: It struck terror in my heart," Mrs. Roseberry recalls. "I was dumbfounded. I didn't know what it meant."

Chips of paint from the Roseberry house were sent to the state for testing. They were loaded with lead. Tests inside the house showed lead on every stick of wood. Paint dust from the wells of each of the 27 windows was loaded with lead. So was the white chalk that rubbed off the house siding. The paint on the porch rail contained 30 percent lead. Three months after Amanda tested above 40 µg/dl, Mrs. Roseberry thought to ask about her younger daughter, who was born after the family moved into the house. Julianne was 10 months old when she was tested; her blood-lead level was over 70 µg/dl. Local health officials declared the Roseberrys' home to be "uninhabitable" for children under the age of six.

"The estimate to remediate the lead was $30,000," Mrs. Roseberry says. "We didn't have the money, and no one would lend it to us." The Roseberrys abandoned their home and declared bankruptcy. "Overnight we went from happy homeowners to homeless family with two lead-poisoned kids."

What makes the story of the Roseberrys' poisonous porch so tragic is that it need never have happened. The hazards that lead paint poses to infants and children have been known since the beginning of this century.

THE UNITED STATES IGNORES A DEADLY HEALTH THREAT

Doctors at the turn of the century in Australia were grappling with a disease described by one as a "Toxicity of Habitation." It was a disease of children, characterized by stomach cramps, paralysis, pain in the limbs, and convulsions. It was finally identified as lead poisoning, and a doctor at the Brisbane Hospital for Sick Children eventually isolated the source: The children were being poisoned by the sweet-tasting white powder that chalked off house paint. It was the first time that lead poisoning in children was traced to lead house paint. The prime point of exposure? Australia's ubiquitous porches.

That was in 1904. At that time, and for many years after, white lead was an important ingredient in paint. (White lead is not a color, but a substance, lead carbonate.) In fact, the quality of paint was determined by the amount of white lead it contained. The process for producing white lead was developed in Holland and became known as the "Dutch Process." Out of that came paint's most famous brand name, "Dutch Boy."

White lead paint could be tinted any color and was used inside and out for everything from houses and barns to toys and cribs.

By the 1920s, there was a worldwide movement to ban the use of white lead. By the end of that decade, most of Europe had ratified the ban. The United States was certainly aware of the dangers of white lead; in 1923, the eighth edition of *Holt's Diseases of Infancy and Childhood* reported eight cases of childhood lead poisoning "caused in each instance by the child's nibbling and swallowing the paint from his crib or furniture." Seven of the children died. By 1926, it was known that there was a deadly relationship between lead poisoning and pica, "perverted appetite for nonfood items." (Children have been known to eat almost anything: paper, pencils, newspaper, clay, sand, plaster, dirt, and, significantly, paint.) No fewer than fifteen publications that year reported that eating lead paint from toys, furniture, and woodwork was a major hazard to infants and children.

But while Europe was banning white lead, the U.S. National Bureau of Standards was recommending its use in private and public buildings, including schools. Any effort to legislate against lead paint ran into a solid wall of bureaucrats and academics, all supported by money channeled through the Lead Industries Association (LIA).*

For decades the lead industry poured money into public relations. The sheer weight of the paint bucket was touted as the measure of quality. Eagle-Pitcher (paint company) ran advertising asking, "Is there enough LEAD in your paint?" and Dutch Boy, promoting "Lead-Consciousness," asked people to discover the "hundred and one ways in which lead enters into the daily life of everyone" by requesting a copy of Dutch Boy's free publication "The Wonder Book of Lead."

In 1943, the U.S. Office of Education and LIA jointly published a booklet that recommended white lead paint for both farm buildings and the interior surfaces of homes.

In 1946, the Harvard University School of Public Health co-sponsored a Lead Industries Association symposium after a faculty member

---

*For a full history of the lead industry's success in delaying regulation in the United States, read *The Hour of Lead*, published in 1992 by the Environmental Defense Fund.

reminded the deans that LIA members had "consistently been our very good friends." The papers presented and published included one from an LIA executive entitled "Facts and Fallacies Concerning Exposure to Lead."

The lead industry and its friends held off legislation for half a century. By 1971, 200 children a year were dying of lead poisoning. That year, Congress finally passed the Lead-Based Poisoning Prevention Act, restricting residential use of lead paint and coincidentally banning its use on toys and children's furniture.* The restrictions finally went into place in 1977. The United States had finally caught up with Europe, but in the intervening half century millions of tons of lead had been applied to everything from exterior siding and interior woodwork to cribs and toys and Sandra Roseberry's porch railing. In fact, ATSDR's official estimate is three million tons—that's tons of lead, not lead paint.

ATSDR estimates there are 57 million housing units that still contain some amount of lead paint (see table). Fourteen million of them contain lead paint that's flaking or peeling, and almost four million of these are occupied by young children (see box for more information on these units). Homes with chipping or peeling paint pose the highest risk, but every house and apartment that contains leaded paint carries with it a measurable risk to its occupants.

WHEN WAS YOUR HOUSE OR APARTMENT BUILT?

The older your home, the more lead its paint may contain. Lead-based paint manufactured before the 1950s tended to have a higher lead con-

---

According to HUD, 3.8 million housing units with lead paint hazards are occupied by families with children under the age of seven.

- 52 percent house families with an annual income under $30,000.
- 48 percent house families with an annual income over $30,000.
- 53 percent are owner occupied.
- 47 percent are rented.

---

*Marine paint, farm equipment paint, automobile paints, and industrial finishes were not covered by this legislation and *still contain lead*. Young children should never be exposed to these products.

centration than paint made after that. Manufacturers of white lead paints boasted of their high lead content, often containing 50 percent lead (500,000 ppm).

Any house or apartment unit built before World War II is almost certain to contain paint with extraordinarily high concentrations of lead. The use of lead-based interior paint declined during the 1950s. Latex paint is much less likely to contain lead. Almost no paint applied after 1980 contained lead.

The greatest concentration of older homes is in the Northeast, in the areas that were developed earliest. This tempts people in other parts of the country to believe they have no reason to be concerned. But there are older homes everywhere—concentrations of pre-1950 housing are not limited to the East Coast. Census data shows that 74 percent of the housing in San Francisco County and 35 percent in Los Angeles was built before 1950.

WHAT WAS A SELLING POINT IS NOW A MAJOR LIABILITY

Lead-based paints were advertised as "self-cleaning" because the surface of the paint's protective film would gradually break down and

HOW MANY KIDS ARE AT RISK?

CONSTRUCTION DATE*	NO. OF UNITS W/LEAD	NO. OF CHILDREN†
Pre-1940	20,505,000	5,885,000
1940–59	16,141,000	4,632,000
1959–74	5,318,000	1,526,000
Total pre-1975	41,964,000	12,043,000

Source: ATSDR, "Report to Congress," 1988

*Although this table ends with 1974, housing built between 1975 and 1980 may also contain lead paint.

†The estimated numbers of children under the age of seven years living in houses and apartments containing lead-based paint.

turn to powder. The powder would wipe or wash off, taking dirt and stains with it. Outside, every rainstorm left the house sparkling! The paints became known as chalking paint because most houses were painted white, and the powder that rubbed off looked like chalk. Indoors, this paint was used on woodwork, baseboards, and window and door frames to make them easier to keep clean.

Lead chalk is easy to see if the paint is white and you rub your hand across it. But if the rain washes it into the soil around the perimeter of the house or it is brushed off a wall to join the dust on the floor, it is invisible. This is extremely dangerous! When children play in that soil, the dirt gets on their hands and into their mouths. (Read chapter 5 for details on lead in soil.) When they inhale lead dust, they are at greatest risk because the dust is so readily absorbed through the lungs.

Lead dust can be recirculated into the air inadvertently by sweeping or vacuuming (the filterbags in household vacuum cleaners are not fine enough to trap lead dust) or simply by people or pets moving through the room. Frequent mopping with a lead-binding detergent is very important in households where lead paint is present (see box, pp. 22–23).

Young children who spend time in a room painted with lead paint are bound to ingest some lead. Lead dust gets on a child's bottle nipple or pacifier when it falls on the floor, or on toys, or on the child's hands while crawling and playing. The items or the child's hands wind up in her mouth.

Some ingestion is deliberate, since a toddler's exploration of the world around her is not limited to what she can see or hear or feel; she also explores taste. And lead chalk tastes sweet. Children like the taste of the white stuff on their hands; some have been found licking paint chalk directly off the side of a house.

Others eat the paint itself. Teething kids chew anything they can get their mouths on. Hundreds of children died in the first half of this century because they chewed crib rails painted with white lead paint. Crib rails don't have lead paint today, but windowsills do, and they're the perfect height and shape for toddlers to get their teeth on. If the paint is in poor condition, chipping and flaking, the teething child is going to get a mouthful of lead.

How much lead does it take to poison a child? Not much. Tom Spitler of the Boston regional office of the EPA translates ppm's and µg/mg's into something we can more readily understand. (The abbreviation mg stands for milligrams.) Think about the amount of salt someone might put on a piece of steak. If that sprinkle of salt was dirt or dust contaminated with just 1,000 ppm lead and a child ate it every day, the child would suffer low-level lead poisoning. Much lead contamination is significantly higher. And most young children eat 50 to 100 mg of dirt every day. Just about enough to salt your steak.

The report of an elevated blood-lead level is a double whammy. The most precious thing in your life, your child, is endangered. Then, as you're dealing with the threat to your child, you realize that your home, your most valuable possession, is also at risk. The degree to which your home is contaminated will determine whether you can stay in it. The Roseberry family lost their home. They are not alone; the cost of lead-paint remediation can easily outstrip your personal finances including the net worth of your home. Remediation does not necessarily mean the removal of lead paint. There are other ways to make the lead less accessible to children, as we'll discuss later in the book.

This realization hit my wife, Andrea, and me like a one-two punch. Our panic over Matthew's condition had barely been quelled when the implications of possible lead-paint contamination hit.

We had fallen in love with our house the instant we saw it. It's a Brooklyn brownstone type (though made of brick), built around 1908, with 10-foot ceilings, ornate plaster, and parquet floors. What really sold us was the fact that no one in the intervening decades had "modernized" it; all the original woodwork was still there. The pocket doors, the wide moldings with ornate lintels framing doors and windows, the built-in cupboards and shelves, the carved mantels, and the giant framed mirror-seat in the living room — all were still in place. And all thickly painted.

Like everyone else, we had to stretch our finances to buy the house. We were still scraping paint and patching plaster on the first floor when the stock market crashed, and home values dropped 25 percent in a wink. When we found out about our son's condition, we couldn't have sold the house if we tried. Yet, the woodwork that we loved so much began to seem menacing every time we walked into a room. I had nightmares in which I was tearing out every stick of trim in the house — that was before I learned how dangerous renovation can be. We were panicking. We knew we had no time to lose in locating and dealing with the lead-paint hot spots in our house.

LOCATING THE SOURCES OF LEAD-PAINT CONTAMINATION

The first thing to do if your child's test shows lead poisoning is to survey your home for lead-paint sources. You're trying to locate the sources of contamination so you can keep your child away from them until they can be eliminated.

You can do this yourself . . . you don't need official paint testing yet. Start by observing carefully where your child spends time. If your child is still an infant, pay close attention to the nursery and any place where the infant may be placed while awake. Is the crib close to a windowsill or other painted surface? Is the crib itself (or anything else the baby may spend time in) old enough to have lead paint on it? Does the baby chew on anything that's painted?

If your child is a toddler, your investigation needs to be more wide-ranging. Look at every painted surface the child touches or that could be shedding lead-paint dust onto the floor where the child plays. Don't stop at the front door; if your child plays on a porch, as Amanda Roseberry did, or near other exterior paint, you'll want to look at that too.

What are you looking for? Cracking or chipping or flaking paint.

- Check for paint chips or granules on the floor.

- Window wells—the space where the sash fits between the window sill and the storm-screen—are usually hotbeds of lead.

- Look for paint-chip or dust accumulation.

- Look for loose paint that a child could flake off.

- Look especially for signs that painted objects are being chewed.

- Windowsills and furniture—which the child can get his mouth around—should be one of the first places to look.

- Check metal objects; radiators and iron railings and gates are often sources of lead-paint chips. Look behind radiators; paint that's close to heat often cracks and peels.

- Rub your hand over painted surfaces, especially outdoors. If your hand picks up a chalky powder, you've isolated a problem.

- If your house has clapboard siding, check the bottom edge of the clapboards; they're often peeling even when the front surface is in good shape.

You may not find much. You're trying to eliminate the obvious. You'll probably find routine nicks and dings in the woodwork, and perhaps a spot or two that's peeling, but unless your child's blood-lead levels are approaching Class III (see chapter 2), you aren't likely to uncover significant sources of lead-paint exposure. But be aware that this does not eliminate paint as a potential source of lead poisoning, since lead-paint dust is invisible.

With one exception, the paint in our house was in good shape—not cracking or peeling. Andrea and I immediately dealt with the exception. The house still had all of its original wooden venetian blinds, loaded with who knows how many layers of paint. Every time a breeze blew in the window, the blinds would chatter and shed a dusting of paint chips on the floor below. The blinds came down the day we got Matthew's test results.

Just as we needed reassurance about Matthew's condition, we needed information about how sick our house was. I went to the hardware store and bought a kit to test for lead paint (see box, pp. 43–44). I broke the little vials and squeezed and rubbed, but I frankly couldn't tell whether the indicator had changed color or I was just looking for it to change. We needed something more conclusive.

We learned that because Matthew's lead level was over 20 μg/dl, we could call the New York City Health Department and get a free lead-paint test. (This was in 1991; local health officials are now notified automatically of all elevated lead levels, and New York law now requires health inspectors to make on-premise lead inspections whenever lead levels over 20 μg/dl are reported.)

Olga Fernandez showed up with a bag of equipment, a clipboard with a full-page checklist, and an armful of literature. We got a quick lesson in how children are exposed to lead paint, and our house got a thorough physical. Before she was done, she had collected a water sample, a soil sample, and two dust samples and had used a portable X-ray machine to measure for lead at 27 different locations. Four of them were positive.

Ms. Fernandez stalked our house like a latter-day Sherlock Holmes; her hi-tech magnifying glass let her "see" through layers of paint to identify where the dreaded lead was hiding. She worked with a handheld XRF—for X-ray fluorescence—machine. She would hold the machine against a painted surface, click it, and have an instant reading; she was x-raying our paint! (More on XRF testing on pp. 46–47.)

She moved quickly through the house. Although lead was more often used in shiny enamel paints than in flat wall paint, that doesn't preclude lead being found on plaster walls and even ceilings. But the

DO-IT-YOURSELF TESTING FOR
LEAD PAINT

There are a number of do-it-yourself test kits available to help you look for lead paint. They are best used for preliminary screening.

Most kits are multipurpose testing tools, good for paint, ceramics, solder—almost anything solid—but they cannot be used to test water.

The home tests will tell you if high levels of lead are present, but they don't tell you how much lead is present, and their accuracy in testing low levels of lead is uncertain.

Their advantage is they are inexpensive, and you get results instantaneously. When they are used to test ceramics, you don't have to break the dish to test it. (It may seem silly, but some lab tests for ceramic lead require a broken dish.)

All use a chemical reagent that changes color when exposed to lead. Sodium sulfide is most commonly used; it turns dark brown or black in the presence of lead. Other kits use a reagent that turns pink. The kits have a shelf life of about a year, although you have no idea how long a kit has been sitting on the shelf before you buy it. Most require you to mix two chemicals to make the test solution. Once mixed, the solution is good for four to six weeks if properly stored.

The problem I had using the home-test kit was that I was testing only the top layer of paint. Lead paint went off the market more than 15 years ago. There's a good chance in any house that's been maintained that the lead-based paint has been painted over. Certainly the really bad pre-1950 stuff has been painted over. Researching this book, I collected instructions for every kit I could find; most recommend cutting through the layers of paint down to the original surface with a knife to expose the old lead. One kit, certainly the most complete, includes a razor blade and suggests cutting on the bias or diagonal so the various paint layers are more exposed; it also includes a small magnifying glass for examining the layers for color change.

Since the test kits depend on color change, they work best on white or light-colored paints. Looking for dark brown or dark gray on a dark paint can get pretty subjective. Some reagents react to other nontoxic heavy metals (titanium) that may be in paint, possibly giving a false positive, and some cannot be used on iron radiators and railings.

For paint, home-test kits would seem to have limited use for initial screening. They are no substitute for professional lead-paint testing. Appendix H includes specific information on a number of home-test kits, including ordering information.

If you have a lead-poisoned child, you may be able to get your home inspected for lead paint at no cost by contacting your local health or environmental agency or housing authority.

Some states offer a similar testing program. See appendix D for a listing of state lead program contacts.

There are many private companies that will test paint for lead. They may use XRF in the home or test paint samples in the lab or both. You should be able to get a list of certified inspection companies either from local health officials or from your state contact.

Since XRF testing is done in the home, there usually is a minimum charge. The total charge depends on the number of spots tested. Figure from $30 to $75 a room.

Laboratories charge anywhere from $15 to as much as $70 per sample to test chips you send them. Having a technician come to your house to collect the chip samples will add another $100 to $200.

PROFESSIONAL TESTING

You should be prepared to ask a lot of questions if you plan to hire a private company to test for lead paint:

■ Have workers completed an EPA training course?

■ How complete will the survey be? Windows and doors, of course, but all woodwork? And walls? How about painted kitchen and/or bathroom cabinets? How many samples will be taken?

■ What method will be used? XRF, lab test, or combination?

■ Is the company certified? By whom?

■ How much information will you get? Written report? Positive/negative or actual readings?

■ How much will the entire survey cost?

more likely places are windows, doors, wood trim, and all surfaces in kitchens and baths. Our house has forced air heat, but she explained that the iron radiators used with steam and hot-water systems are often loaded with lead paint—and frequently overlooked. So are the pipes you sometimes find in the corner of a room, carrying hot water or steam to upper floors. Also wrought iron rails and gates on porches and steps.

Clear finishes may also contain lead. Lead acetate, also known as "Sugar of Lead" for its sweet taste, was used as a drier in old varnish. If your toddler runs her hand down the stairwell bannister, the finish on it should be checked for lead.

Ms. Fernandez paid special attention to window frames and sashes, explaining that a fine layer of window paint is ground off every time the window is opened and closed. Even though the paint on the windows tested negative for lead, she took a sample of the dust in one window well to make sure powdered lead wasn't blowing in from outside.

She was done in less than an hour. Two floors, three bedrooms, hallway, kitchen, bath and a half . . . and a long form filled out. Health Department Agent Fernandez found lead paint in one room in our house—the small hallway between Matthew's bedroom and the bath. With all the woodwork in our home, the worst lead paint she found was on three tiny plaster walls, one bedroom door, and the bathroom door frame.

The offending surfaces were stamped with an indelible purple-ink condemnation stamp, a warning that they were contaminated with lead paint and must be removed.

I may be the first person in the world to feel this way, but I thought those purple stamps were the most beautiful things I'd ever seen because they signaled that we had exposed the enemy and we had it cornered; the lead paint was limited to just a tiny part of our house. Best of all, it was one of the few places where we hadn't already worked. Had we gotten to the little foyer and started patching and sanding there, the lead dust would have spread throughout our home. We counted ourselves very lucky.

A couple of weeks after our inspection, we received a notice from the city. Our purple-stamped items were official lead poisoning violations under the New York City Health Code. The letter informed us we had ten days to start remediation, or the city would start it for us—and fine us! Continued violation could result in a jail sentence of up to one year! We didn't need to be forced to comply—we'd already started.

PROS AND CONS OF THE PROFESSIONAL TESTS FOR LEAD PAINT

XRF TESTING

As good as the XRF testing device is, it has serious limitations. As one professional tester told me, if it says there's no lead, there's no lead. And if it says there's a lot of lead, there's a lot of lead. The problem is the gray area in the middle. Using the XRF analyzer is part science, part art; its accuracy is highly dependent on the training, ability, and experience of the technician using it.

The XRF analyzer uses a radioactive source to measure lead in paint. The machine itself has a lead shield inside it, to protect the technician from radiation, but the shield has been known to slip—held in certain positions, the machine starts measuring itself. A sharp technician will notice the discrepancy; a not-so-sharp operator will have you tearing your walls down.

Another problem is that the XRF can't tell where the paint stops and the rest of the house starts. A testing supervisor in Pennsylvania related a case where an XRF test showed a painted wall to be loaded with lead. Nothing else in the house tested positive, so he went back to doublecheck the measurements. He found the hot spot, but when he moved the XRF to either side, he found no lead. Going back to the hot spot, he moved the XRF up and down, and traced a vertical line of lead on the wall. "There was no lead in that paint," he said. "There was an old lead pipe behind the plaster."

An advantage to using XRF is it doesn't require removing paint samples, so you don't face a major patching job once the test is done. It's relatively inexpensive, and you get the results immediately. But XRF requires experience and interpretation. And even with that, lead levels that fall in the gray area should be verified with laboratory analysis of paint chips before you start ripping out woodwork. Experts don't agree on what the boundaries of the gray area are, but for its public housing, New York City requires lab verification of direct XRF readings between .04 and 1.0 mg/cm^2 (milligrams per square centimeter). The state of Maryland recommends laboratory confirmation for readings between 0.5 and 2.0 mg/cm^2.

LABORATORY ANALYSIS

The definitive test for lead in paint is atomic absorption laboratory analysis of paint chips. This involves removing a sample of paint from every surface to be tested. You don't need to worry about getting an unbroken piece of paint; the sample will be ground up in the lab before being tested. The sample should be about one square inch and must include all layers of paint. (Agent Fernandez used her XRF machine to test 27 spots for lead in our house; had we scraped paint from each of those spots, we'd have been left with the house looking like it had a bad case of pox.) Another concern is how you collect those samples; removing multiple layers of paint like that is certain to generate tiny chips and dust. It's important to carry a spray bottle of water with you as you scrape off the sample of paint. Spray and wipe as you work, to keep the dust down and to catch as many particles as you can.

You can get laboratory results in 24 to 48 hours. Paint containing lead levels of more than 0.5 percent by weight in a dried solid form is considered to be lead paint. Lead content may also be expressed as 5,000 mg/km (milligrams per kilogram). For more than a few samples, laboratory testing for lead in paint can become very expensive.

The sensible thing to do is to get an XRF test to screen for lead and then send chips to a laboratory to verify any readings that are inconclusive. You don't need to replicate every test; if you get 15–20 readings all around 0.9–1.1, scrape paint off three or four scattered locations. If they are all confirmed to be lead paint, you can be confident that the other spots are too. Of course, if the XRF screening shows isolated hot spots of lead paint, you may decide, as we did, to simply go ahead and deal with the problem.

It is very important that you not begin removing known or suspected lead paint without taking extensive precautions (see chapter 4). Removal may not be the best or even the most practical remedy. Improper removal of lead paint may release lethal levels of lead dust into your home. In dealing with either a contractor or an inspector, ask if they're following the new HUD guidelines, and ask to see a copy.

4

REMODELING, REPAINTING, AND ABATEMENT

The paint falls—you know, they're redoing the White House—and she's licking her feet and she's ingested lead.

> *—Then-President George Bush, announcing that Presidential Spaniel Millie was diagnosed as lead poisoned*

WHAT GEORGE BUSH didn't tell reporters when he revealed Millie's malady was that government experts were warning the president against allowing his many grandchildren to visit or play in the White House as long as the renovations continued. It's unfortunate the President missed a golden opportunity to focus national attention on the high risk faced by children during lead-paint renovations. There's no telling how many cases of childhood lead poisoning could have been prevented had the president passed the health warnings he was getting on to the public.

Millie was not the first dog to be lead poisoned during the renovation of an old home; she was just the most famous. A sickened pet is often the first warning a family gets that there is a deadly poison in the home. Dogs are as notorious as kids for chewing and eating almost anything. Both dogs and cats groom themselves by licking, thus exposing themselves to the deadly lead dust released by remodeling and renovation. Without meaning to do so, they serve as sentinels for their families.

THE CASE OF THE POISONED TERRIER

Veterinarian Gregory Bayan has seen five cases of lead-poisoned dogs in the eleven years he's been in practice. The mixed-breed terrier that came into the Rhinebeck, New York, Animal Hospital was typical, he says, brought in because it had tremors or the shakes, and was very weak. He ran a blood count, and the test showed elevated levels of nucleated red blood cells without anemia, a "red flag" of lead poisoning.

Dr. Bayan asked if the dog had had any exposure to lead. The dog's owner explained that her home was undergoing extensive renovation, with layers of old paint being scraped and sanded off the walls, ceilings, doors, molding, and even the old painted floors. The woman said the dog was particularly fond of one of the workmen and often sat at his feet while he was sanding. The dog would get coated with paint dust and then lick herself clean.

The dog belonged to a young family. The father commuted several hours each day to work in New York City, and traveled on business. The mother worked out of an office in their newly purchased 10-room Victorian farmhouse. This arrangement allowed her to care for their two children, a five-year-old daughter, who attended half-day sessions of kindergarten during the week, and a 20-month-old son.

The family took an extended vacation, from August to mid-September, so as to be out of the house while the renovation work was being done, but the work wasn't finished when they returned. To speed the delayed renovation job along, the mother helped by stripping paint from hallway moldings, using a torch to heat and lift the paint. A babysitter was hired to keep the children out of the way, usually outdoors, while the renovation work continued. The sitter came for five hours a day, five days a week, and brought her own two children, ages two and three, with her.

The dog had become sick in mid-October. The paint dust was on everything, its owner told the veterinarian—on the carpets, the furniture, the children's toys. Dr. Bayan recommended having the children tested for lead poisoning. The vet began chelation therapy on the dog. Two days later, the dog had improved enough to go home, where chelation would continue. But after three days at home, the terrier died.

In the meantime, the family was starting to report various symptoms. The mother was feeling weak and tired. Her daughter complained of stomachaches. The father experienced an episode of severe nausea after spending a weekend at home while paint was being burned off with torches. In early November, the family was tested for lead, first with the FEP test and then with a blood-lead test.

The father, who spent the least amount of time in the house, tested at 33 μg/dl, more than three times the CDC action level and well into Class III lead poisoning. The mother's blood-lead level was 47 μg/dl; the daughter's, 56 μg/dl; and the toddler's, a staggering 87 μg/dl. The mother and her two children were immediately admitted to a local hospital, and chelation treatment was begun on all three.

The chelating drug was administered for five days, followed by a two-day break. The daughter required three week-long cycles before her blood-lead level was under control; the son underwent chelation for a total of five weeks. Shortly after their family was found to be lead poisoned, the baby-sitter and her two children were tested. Her level was mildly elevated at 18 μg/dl, but her two children's levels were 57 and 67 μg/dl, and the two of them were also hospitalized and chelated.

This story was the subject of a case report in the *American Journal of Public Health,* not because it was unusual but because acute lead poisoning is being found more and more frequently among homesteaders, young professionals with small children living in older homes being renovated and restored. At Children's Hospital in Boston, 30 percent of the infant lead poisoning cases reported between 1987 and 1990 were the result of exposure in an older home that was being renovated.

BE AWARE OF THE DANGERS

HUD is writing a new bible for dealing with lead paint. It's called "Guidelines for the Evaluation and Control of Lead-Based Paint Hazards in Housing." It is available in draft form now, with the final form expected early in 1995. Note the word "hazards" in the title. Significantly, HUD regulations, which ultimately drive housing regulation, are becoming more sophisticated, moving beyond the control of lead paint to the control of the risks the lead paint poses.

The new guidelines recognize the threat posed by lead-paint dust, as evidenced by the poisoning of Millie, the upstate New York family, and countless others. Lead paint, secure or peeling, that is scraped, sanded, or burned off releases enormous quantities of lead into the home environment. Even if the visible chips and scrapings are cleaned up, the home will be filled with lead dust and, in the case of paint that has been heated, lead fumes and vapors. Extensive renovation projects involving lead paint where there is a child present almost always result in acute lead poisoning requiring chelation and/or hospitalization.

Any home improvement project involving a surface coated with lead paint—whether it's as small as sanding a door that binds or as large as sanding the outside of the house—requires special treatment, especially if children are present. For any but the smallest project, children should be removed from the home until the project is complete. As we'll discuss below, that includes special cleaning procedures once the physical work is done.

Don't overreact if you discover that your child has an elevated lead level. Hearing that diagnosis creates all kinds of fears. Fear prompts action. Your first impulse will be to rid your home of lead paint. The danger is that if removal is improperly done, it can vastly *increase* your child's exposure and turn manageable low-level lead poisoning into a case of life-threatening acute toxicity. Shortly after Baltimore became one of the first cities to publicize the dangers of lead paint—in the early 1980s, before the danger of lead-paint dust was known—almost half of the lead poisoning cases treated at the city's Kennedy Krieger Institute were coming from homes where lead paint had been improperly removed.

IF YOU RENT . . .

The discussion of lead-paint abatement in this chapter is primarily of interest to people who own their homes and must take responsibility for lead-paint problems themselves. If you are a renter, you must turn to your landlord for relief. The information in this chapter will help you determine whether your landlord has resolved the problem correctly. (Dealing with a landlord, private or public, is covered in chapter 11.)

SEPARATE YOUR CHILD FROM THE SOURCE OF LEAD

Your responsibility, if testing shows your home to have lead paint, is to assess its risk and then eliminate the paint as a potential or actual source of lead poisoning. You basically have three options:

■ Remove your child from the source of exposure. This may be the simplest—and sometimes your only—short-term solution.

■ Remove the source from your home. This may be as simple as diligent housecleaning or as complex as physically removing paint from all interior and exterior surfaces.

■ Create a physical barrier between your child and the lead paint. Short-term, this could mean closing off a room; long-term, it could mean covering walls with Sheetrock or re-siding the house.

Your mop and bucket are your first line of defense against poisoning from lead paint. Even large chips and visible particles should be picked up with a damp mop. Any dusting, sweeping, or vacuuming is going to stir up lead dust, scattering it further about the home. Follow the directions in chapter 2 for making a washing solution and then use it regularly on all interior surfaces (including furniture) you suspect of bearing lead paint or dust. Pay especial attention to window wells. Washing to remove lead-paint dust doesn't mean wiping with a damp sponge—that just moves the dust around; it means getting the surface really wet and then mopping.

This careful attention to cleaning, coupled with nutritional modifications and the use of bottled water for your child (see chapter 6), may be sufficient to bring and keep your child's lead level below the magic 10 µg/dl even if you have some lead paint in your home. However, this will be true *only* for low-level lead poisoning, and even then, you may wish, as we did, to remove the threat completely. Obviously, any lead paint that is loose, peeling, flaking, or chalking must be abated. Depending on where you live, you may have no choice but to abate all lead-paint hazards.

THE ABATEMENT DILEMMA

There are six steps to the effective abatement of lead paint in a home. The risk of lead poisoning has not been eliminated until all six steps have been successfully completed.

■ Testing—to determine the scope of work needed.
■ Selection—to determine which hazard control technique(s) to use.
■ Containment—to keep from contaminating new areas.
■ Implementation—replacement, encapsulation, and/or removal.
■ Cleaning up—removal of debris and dust.
■ Retesting—to be sure the lead threat is gone.

Abating lead-based paint can be a nightmare. Unless your lead-paint problem is small or your bank account large, you will have to compromise something. Here's the dilemma: To be done properly, abatement can be prohibitively expensive; done improperly, it can be recklessly dangerous. The new HUD guidelines recognize that with lead paint in some 57 million homes, not everyone is going to be able to fully abate the hazard at the time of discovery. HUD makes provisions for "Interim Controls," common sense measures that will reduce the risk of lead-paint poisoning. These recommendations include specialized cleaning, repair and maintenance, painting and temporary containment, and education. Interim measures are always accompanied by on-going monitoring (usually of lead dust) to make sure the measures are working. Parents often face a Hobson's choice, where you're asked to decide between physical health and fiscal health. No one can make your decisions for you. This book can't make them for you. It can, however, give you the facts necessary to make informed decisions. Taking interim measures may be the best you can do. It is certainly better than doing nothing.

Before you consider any abatement work, call your local health department or the number listed in appendix D for your state. Ask what, if any, laws or guidelines apply to lead-paint abatement. Some states or locales have strict laws governing who can do abatement work, how it should be done, and whether you can stay in your home during abatement. Within the next few years, federal law will require abatement contractors to be licensed.

One of the biggest problems confronting families having to deal with lead poisoning and lead paint has been getting good information. Often the very people or sources you would normally turn to for help are uninformed or, even worse, misinformed on the subject of lead paint and lead poisoning.

Marc and Kathryn Perrone carefully researched the best way to remove the lead paint, which was several layers thick, on the woodwork of their early-1900s Milwaukee home. They knew the paint was a threat to their 18-month-old daughter. They finally decided on a method using a heat gun. Before committing to the heat gun, Mrs. Perrone called paint stores and an environmental consulting firm for second opinions. Everyone agreed the heat gun was safe.

Halfway through the work on the hallway, Mrs. Perrone read someplace else that using a heat gun was a dangerous way to remove lead paint. She immediately called her pediatrician. "He completely dismissed me," she says. "He thought it [her concern for her daughter's health] was the silliest thing he'd ever heard." Fortunately, Mrs. Perrone persisted; her daughter's blood-lead level was 33 μg/dl, more than three times the present threshold.

When Anne and Kevin Sheehan renovated the old farmhouse they'd purchased in upstate New York, they did so under the direction of HUD. They paid for the house and renovation with a Federal Housing Authority (FHA) mortgage, which was contingent on making certain repairs to the house, including repainting. HUD officials reviewed without comment a number of work orders, all calling for sanding off the old paint. Indeed, a HUD notification concerning lead-paint poisoning, which the Sheehans were required to sign at the mortgage closing, instructed them that "before repainting, all surfaces that are peeling, chipping or loose should be thoroughly cleaned by washing, sanding or brushing the loose paint from the surface."

The Sheehans sanded. They released so much lead dust that not only was their 30-month-old daughter lead poisoned but their house was so thoroughly contaminated the state of New York ordered them to vacate it. The Sheehans also had trouble getting solid medical advice and ended up traveling to nearby Massachusetts to get their daughter treated. "We were completely frustrated," wrote Mrs. Sheehan, who is editor of the local newspaper, "that there was so little information readily available about lead poisoning except simple lists of healthy foods and potential sources."

When we were trying to learn what to do about the lead paint in our hallway, I got a brochure from the New York State Department of Health entitled "Removing Lead-Based Paints." The first advice it gives is that all lead-based paint accessible to children "should be completely removed by scraping and sanding." It also lists gas-fired torches as a way to remove paint but says only experienced people should do this because of the "extreme fire hazard potential." Any one of the three—scraping, sanding, or open-flame burning—would have significantly raised Matthew's exposure to lead poisoning.

HUD has come a long way since its dealings with the Sheehans, and is now taking a leadership role. Recognizing both the costs and problems associated with lead-paint abatement, the new HUD guidelines are in essence establishing a new profession, that of lead-paint risk assessor. More than an inspector, the assessor goes into a dwelling, identifies the presence of lead paint, and then assesses the risk the paint poses before recommending what remedial steps be taken. Unfortunately, while the federal government has moved beyond automatically demanding removal of all lead paint, state and local governments lag far behind. You may find yourself ordered to take actions that could actually increase the risk to your family.

PROPER VERSUS PRAGMATIC APPROACHES TO THE PROBLEM

If testing shows that you have a major lead-paint hazard, you should call in a qualified contractor. Projects involving lead paint, whether renovation, remodeling, or abatement, are not typical do-it-yourself projects. They require special knowledge and special equipment. The risks are high, and the consequences of failure, significant. If not done properly, lead-paint abatement will increase the risk to you and your children. It can also create a situation that will be vastly more expensive to remedy than the original abatement would have been.

But professional lead-paint abatement is expensive. The Perrones, whose house has aluminum siding, called in a contractor to remove the lead paint from the exterior wood trim. The estimate was $10,000, "so far out of our range," Kathryn says, "we didn't know what to do." For many families, the cost of lead abatement exceeds not only what they have in the bank but also the equity they have in the house. Families often find they can't even arrange a loan to have the work done.

Andrea and I did the abatement work in our hallway ourselves. Between a new baby and a new house, there wasn't much money left, and it was a small job in a confined area. Is this recommended? No. Did we make mistakes? Yes, but fortunately, we had done enough research that our mistakes were not costly, either in money or in health.

Sweat equity is a great American tradition; it's the only way many of us can afford our homes. You may find you have no choice but to do some or even all of the work yourself. The information presented here is designed to help you minimize risk and exposure, whether you contract the work out or do it yourself. But please understand that you undertake any project involving lead paint *at your own risk*.

The proper way to deal with any lead-paint problem of significance is to move out of your house or apartment while a qualified contractor does the abatement work. This is the only way to truly minimize both short- and long-term risk.

As the Sheehans and many others have learned, if the lead-paint contamination in a home is serious enough, health officials won't give you an option; they'll declare your home unfit for habitation and order you to move. If you're in an apartment, the landlord may be required to provide alternative housing. But if you own your home, this is a double whammy. Not only do you face the cost of abatement, you have to find—and pay for—a place to live while continuing to keep up your mortgage. The Sheehans were out of their home for two and a half years before health officials declared it sufficiently abated that they could move back in (and they're now living on one floor while cleanup continues on the other).

Although it is best to move out while the work is done, this option may not be open to you, and so we'll explore alternate ways to achieve the desired end. If you are contemplating a remodeling, renovation, or abatement project, your concern is to limit the exposure of adults and older children and *eliminate exposure for pregnant women and children under the age of seven.* How you handle this challenge depends in part on the size and immediacy of the job and in part on your circumstances. Some considerations:

■ If you are buying a home, have the work involving lead paint done before you move in. Beginning in October 1995, you will have 10 days in which to have a new home tested, and the seller must inform you of any known lead that's present.

■ If your present home needs lead-paint work and you can afford or arrange (by staying with relatives, for example) to move out, by all means do so.

■ If you cannot move the entire family out, children under the age of seven should be sent to live elsewhere until the work, including cleanup, is complete. The younger the child, the more imperative this is. Children under 30 months are at greatest risk.

■ It's not enough to keep children out of the home while work is being done during the day. The threat comes from the dust generated during the project; the home is not safe for children until it has been thoroughly cleaned.

■ *Under no circumstances should a child who has been treated for lead poisoning be returned to the home until the source of lead has been completely abated.*

■ If you are not dealing with an immediate lead-paint hazard, and you're removing paint only for aesthetic reasons, consider putting the work off until your children are older. "Weigh your child's health versus the aesthetics of fine woodwork," says Kathryn Perrone. "Nothing is worth your child's health."

■ Schedule the work around summer vacations when your family is away, or at least ship the kids to visit relatives.

■ Work on one floor, live on the other.

■ Work on one room at a time. The same concept as above. Both of these alternatives require careful attention to containment to make sure that dust and debris are not tracked from the work area to the living area. Be compulsive about washing—your hands, pacifiers and nipples, toys, the rest of the home.

Another way to limit exposure is to limit the amount of work you do. If you're not required by law to abate all lead-painted surfaces, consider selective abatement. Windows, with their abrasive up-and-down movement, are prime generators of lead dust. At the same time, windows old enough to carry lead paint are often loose and poorly insulated. Window replacement will not only remove a major lead-paint threat but also cut future heating costs. Doors also generate lead dust through friction; they can be sent out to be stripped. If you're dealing with a low-level lead poisoning situation, these actions may be sufficient to reduce your child's exposure enough to bring blood-lead levels below the 10 µg/dl level.

HIRING A CONTRACTOR

Finding a qualified contractor can be a challenge. Start with your local health department; it may have a list of recommended firms. If that fails, call the state lead contact listed in appendix D or your regional HUD office (listed in appendix E).

Jot down questions as you read this chapter and be prepared to ask them. You need to know a lot more than just what the contractor will do and what the job will cost; just as important is how the contractor will do the work, what precautions workers will take, and how well they'll clean up after the work is done. The threat from lead-paint poisoning is not gone until, literally, the dust is cleared.

Try to locate a contractor who has been through a lead abatement training program and is certified. It's difficult to find certified contractors right now but should become easier as Title X requirements for state certification kick in over the next one to two years. The potential growth of lead-paint removal as an industry is evidenced by the existence of the National Lead Abatement Council, which, among other things, publishes *Deleading*, a bimonthly magazine. Appendix L lists regional EPA sanctioned training centers. Training in lead-paint abatement is open to anyone, including do-it-yourselfers who want to handle their lead-paint problems themselves.

Start with the recommendations of the lead-risk assessor as your guide. Always talk to—and get quotes from—more than one contractor. Try to get quotes for different methods of abatement. A knowledgeable lead-paint abatement contractor will usually propose using a number of different techniques, and different contractors may recommend different solutions. You need to be fully informed by the time you begin these discussions.

Within the next year, any contractor undertaking remodeling or renovation work will be required by law to give you a copy of an EPA booklet called "Lead Based Paint—Protect Your Family." (The exact timing of this is uncertain; it depends on the EPA's drafting of worker certification standards, and the agency is behind schedule.) The law will cover anyone doing painting, wallpapering, floor stripping, window replacement, siding, and numerous small projects as well as full-scale renovation projects. The fact that a contractor gives you the EPA booklet does not mean the EPA approves his work or that he is certified.

CONTAINMENT—DON'T MAKE THINGS WORSE

Any project involving lead paint must start with containment. Inside or out, you want to remove the contamination, not spread it. Remember that lead-paint dust (and fumes, if you use a heat gun) are far more dangerous than the large paint chips that are easy to see and simple to remove. The more attention that's paid to containing lead-paint debris and dust, the easier it will be to clean up once the work is done.

Start by removing all furniture and other movable items from the work area. Remove all window treatments and carpeting before work starts; a carpet that is already contaminated should be wet down before being removed. Even if you plan to replace the carpet after the work is finished, take it up now because removing carpet after the work is done will release enormous clouds of lead dust, in and out of your home. Draperies should probably be replaced; it's very difficult to remove lead dust from them. Cover nonremovable items like radiators with 6-mil plastic and seal with duct tape. If you have forced-air heat or central air-conditioning, be sure to cover and seal intakes and vents. If abatement is to be done in the kitchen, *all* food, dishes, pots and pans, utensils, and anything else to do with food must be removed.

The floor needs to be covered and sealed so paint dust doesn't fill the cracks between floorboards. Old floors act as reservoirs, collecting lead dust which is then released every time you walk through the room. Lay down and tape either heavy-duty plastic or construction paper. Use a double layer to protect against tears and make cleanup easier.

The room or work area also needs to be sealed off. Don't just close doors; cover the doorways—and windows—with plastic and tape. This makes for a hot, sticky, dirty, uncomfortable job. If it's stifling, and a window has to be opened, loosely cover the outside to direct the air down, and place a fabric drop cloth saturated with your washing solution on the ground underneath. You want to avoid contaminating the soil outside your home with lead (see chapter 5). Do not run a fan in an area where lead paint is being removed.

Containment when stripping paint from the outside of a building is more of a challenge. The solution is to draw inspiration from the artist Christo and drape the building. Tom Spitler, who is a senior research scientist with the EPA's regional office in Boston, recently had the exterior of his 40-year-old cedar-shake-sided house sandblasted—a once-and-for-all solution, he says. His contractor sunk posts about six feet out from the house and erected a fence of plastic sheeting. The ground and plantings were covered with drop cloths, and the sand/lead-paint mix was completely contained. Spitler says setting up the containment took much longer than the removal—sandblasting his house took about an hour a side—but the job was still faster and less expensive than hand-scraping.

The rule of thumb for exterior containment is to cover the ground going out from the foundation three feet for each story being abated, always covering a minimum of five feet out. In other words, for a two-story house, cover the ground six feet out on the sides, nine feet out on the peak-ends.

Containment extends to the people doing the abatement. Workers should wear coveralls, which should be removed before leaving the work area. Shoes should be covered with disposable booties, which also should be taken off before leaving the work area. For their own safety, workers should wear respirators—those white dust masks with the elastic band are no protection against lead dust. Hands (and any other part of the body that was not completely covered the whole time) should be washed thoroughly when leaving the work area.

I know this is a long way from college kids scraping away on ladders in cutoffs and sneakers, but it's time to start dealing with lead as the deadly toxin that it is. As I write this, there are ladders against two houses in the three blocks between my house and the subway station. Men are scraping 70 years of peeling lead-based paint from porches and overhangs with just a couple of drop cloths under their ladders. There are paint chips everywhere—on the porches, on the sidewalks, in the yards, in the neighbor's yards—and this is a street filled with young children. It is maddening to see what we are doing, what could so easily be prevented.

YOUR ABATEMENT OPTIONS

There are a number of different methods for abating lead paint. Every abatement situation has to be analyzed to see which method makes the most sense and is most cost-effective. Those that create the least dust are the safest. Most abatement projects for severe or extensive contamination will typically use different methods in combination.

Replacement is often the easiest, safest, and least expensive way to remove lead paint that's on wood trim. Our 3-by-10-foot hallway that was the lead-paint hot spot has six doorways and an unbelievable amount of wood molding. Not wanting to be stripping paint so close to the baby's room, we planned to remove the molding, send it out to be stripped, and then reinstall it. The quote was out of sight! We did some shopping and located replica molding at a specialty lumber store. Despite paying a premium for the molding, it was cheaper to replace with new than to try to save the old. Replacing the door frames was even more cost effective.

As mentioned earlier, replacing window units, which are labor-intensive to strip, gives you the added benefit of eliminating the heat loss associated with loose sashes and nonthermal glass. It may also be more economical to replace doors, depending on their quality.

Encapsulation, covering the lead paint, is often the most practical and economical way to deal with large surface areas, both inside and outside. Lead-painted ceilings are easy to Sheetrock over. New Sheetrock or paneling can be installed over old plaster walls, and paneling can be installed over painted wainscotting. Both of these jobs require that door and window moldings be shimmed out to reflect the additional wall thickness. Cracks, between sheets of paneling and between molding and Sheetrock, should be caulked to completely isolate the old lead paint and its incumbent dust.

Check your local ordinances before starting any exterior abatement projects. If you live in a historic district, you may not be allowed to replace ornamental wood, and encapsulation with vinyl or aluminum siding will likely be prohibited. When Hurricane Hugo hit Charleston, South Carolina, floodwaters caused a plague of peeling paint. Abatement options were limited because much of Old Charleston is a historic district.

Covering lead paint does not mean simply painting over it with latex or lead-free paint. Abating lead paint by covering it means putting a permanent barrier between the lead paint and your family. New paint is not a permanent barrier. It wears off, exposing the old lead paint. And if the old paint film is starting to weaken, new paint won't keep it from peeling. The lead paint will still be exposed and released into the environment.

Wallpapering is recommended by the EPA as a way to reduce lead-paint exposure, but you must recognize that even vinyl wallcoverings are much less permanent than new Sheetrock or even paneling. Wallpaper can buy you time until your children get past age seven and are not as vulnerable to lead. There is, however, the danger that significant amounts of lead-paint dust will be released if someone else, unaware there's lead-paint underneath, goes to scrape the wallpaper off.

We had planned to cover the lead paint on the walls by Sheetrocking over the plaster, but the walls were in poor condition, and a lot of plaster fell off the wall when the door moldings were removed. We ended up replacing the plaster walls with Sheetrock. You'll appreciate good containment if you do the same; a plaster wall generates a great deal of dust when it comes down!

A better solution, especially if your walls are rough, or if you want to wallpaper over painted paneling, is to resurrect the old practice of hanging a liner first. Canvas liners are traditional and can be either painted or papered over. Polyester liners are available from several sources in varying thicknesses, but not all polyesters can be painted over. For real permanency, you may prefer to use fiberglass liners, which can be painted or papered over. (See appendix G for a list of sources.)

Encapsulant coatings are another way to cover lead paint. These special liquid coatings are an attractive option because they go on like paint—they can be applied with brush, roller, or sprayer—but they can fail if used in the wrong situation or applied improperly. Selecting the proper encapsulant takes professional guidance. Some form a soft, pliable film, while others dry hard. Some form vapor barriers. A few are reinforced by having a woven mat embedded in the first of two coats. Encapsulants are available for interior and exterior use. All of them require proper surface preparation, and the integrity of liquid encapsulants depends heavily on the condition of the material they'll be covering. (See appendix G for a list of sources.)

Maryland, which is a leader in lead-paint abatement, requires preliminary inspection and testing before approval is given to use an encapsulant coating. The purpose of the inspection is to see if liquid encapsulation is even possible. If the job is a candidate, a test patch is applied, and an inspector tests the adhesion and strength of the coating. Even if the job is approved, and then carried out, it must be examined by a state inspector every three months for a full year to make sure the encapsulation hasn't failed.

Floors painted with lead-based paint can be covered with linoleum, sheet-vinyl, ceramic tile, stone, or new wood flooring. Carpeting does nothing to isolate the hazard and in fact is often a reservoir of lead dust.

Outside, aluminum or vinyl siding can cover chalking lead paint on walls. Window frames can also be aluminum or vinyl clad, but that doesn't solve the problem of lead paint on the window itself.

Removal of lead paint is the first thing most people think of; it's probably the last thing they should consider. Removing lead paint generates the most debris and dust. It can involve the use of caustic and dangerous chemicals. It's time-consuming, labor intensive, and expensive to have done professionally. It's a tempting do-it-yourself project, and it's fraught with danger.

If you must go this route, look for items that can be sent out to be commercially stripped. We sent a number of expensive multipaneled solid wood doors from our hallway project to a local dip-n-strip company. They came back quite clear of paint and with only limited raising of the grain. Look for an immersion stripper who uses solvents (such as DMF) as opposed to lye. Lye is very caustic, will raise a lot of grain, and can dissolve glue joints as well as paint. If you have veneer doors (instead of solid wood), ask the stripping company if their chemicals will delaminate the veneer. If they say no, get it in writing!

Doors, mantles, large cornices, radiators, and both interior and exterior shutters are prime candidates for commercial stripping. If you have unusual molding or trim that can be removed but can't be replaced, it may pay to remove it, send it out for stripping, and then reinstall it. As you remove each piece, mark it so you know where to return it. Ask the stripping company for advice on a marking product that will survive paint stripper.

Sometimes, lead-based paint has to be removed in place, either in preparation for another form of abatement or as a final remedy. A number of tools and methods are available:

Wet scraping is used to remove chipping, loose, or peeling paint prior to encapsulation. It can also be used to completely denude small sections of lead paint but is not practical for large areas of work. The painted surface is constantly and thoroughly wetted using a garden mister with a lead-binding solution to reduce the release of dust while the surface is scraped.

Caustic or chemical strippers line the shelves of paint stores. They're available as liquids, gels, and pastes, flammable and non-flammable, water wash and solvent wash, but most are toxic or hazardous to use. Methylene chloride strippers are by far the most effective, but their fumes can cause kidney damage, irregular heartbeats, and even heart attacks. A proper respirator is essential. The new non-volatile strippers are safer (for humans and the environment), but they're painfully slow, often requiring an overnight application before lifting paint.

The CDC warns that when used on porous surfaces such as wood or stone, chemical strippers leave a residue of lead that is difficult or impossible to clean. This method is considered inadequate for such items as window sashes and doors which have surfaces that rub. Maryland and some other states do not allow the use of methylene chloride.

When working with any chemical that can lift paint, take the following precautions:

■ Wear neoprene gloves to protect your hands. Dishwashing gloves would be dissolved by some chemicals.
■ Wear goggles to protect your eyes.
■ Wear a long-sleeved shirt and pants to protect your skin.
■ Use an approved respirator to keep from breathing harmful vapors. Dust masks will *not* protect you.
■ Follow carefully all directions on the can or packaging.

HEPA sanders incorporate a vacuum to lift the dust generated by sanding and carry it into a HEPA filter bag. A HEPA filter will catch lead dust; regular bag-sanders will not. HEPA sanders are useful only on flat surfaces. They are most useful on floors. *No other kind of sander should be used on lead paint.* If a contractor is going to sand lead paint in your home, make him show you the plate on the machine that says it has HEPA filtration. HEPA stands for High Efficiency Particle Air, and it refers to a filter capable of removing particles down to 0.3 micron in diameter from the air passing through it. It must do that with 99.97 percent efficiency.

Electric heat guns are useful on thick layers of paint on flat surfaces. However, as the Perrone family discovered, heat guns can generate lead fumes as well as dust. Since heat guns blow hot air on the painted surface, they blow lead dust all over the place. Workers must wear special respirators designed to block lead fumes, and no one else should be in the home when this type of work is being done. Heat gun removal usually has to be followed with chemical stripping. Heat guns do not work on metal surfaces.

Blasting paint off, whether with sand or water, is often the most efficient way to deal with exterior paint. This is clearly not an undertaking for an amateur; your primary concern when discussing this option with a contractor is how the waste—sand/paint or water/paint— will be contained and disposed of.

CLEANING UP: THE OTHER HALF OF THE JOB

Lead paint has not been fully abated until all of it is out of harm's way. That includes the cleanup and removal of all debris, large and small. Removing lead paint generates hazardous waste, and proper cleanup starts with the safe bagging and removal of all lead-paint waste. The debris from cleaning a single home can, in most locales, legally be disposed of as household waste (to end up in a municipal or lined landfill), but it must be done carefully. You don't want to go to the trouble and expense of removing lead from your home only to spill it in your yard. The Maryland Division of Lead Poisoning Prevention recommends using 6-mil plastic bags or double-bagging 4-mil garbage bags.

Contaminated materials include any wood or plaster actually removed, the sludge and liquid waste generated by stripping and cleaning, sponges, mop heads, rags, HEPA filters used for cleanup, drop cloths, even gloves and disposable coveralls worn during the project. Large painted objects, windows for instance, should be wrapped in 6-mil plastic drop cloths and sealed with duct tape before being taken out of the removal area. Make sure that lead-contaminated debris is kept away from children or animals until it is removed from the site.

Never burn lead-paint debris. Burning releases lead fumes, the most easily absorbed form of lead, and the remaining ash, highly toxic, will pollute the environment. For the same reason, don't pour liquid lead-bearing waste into a storm sewer or onto the ground.

The work area—as well as any area that has been exposed to lead-paint dust—must now be cleaned. Cleaning is done with a special HEPAvac—essentially a fancy vacuum cleaner capable of lifting and trapping the minute particles of lead dust. HEPAvacs may be available through tool rental centers, or your local public health department may have one to lend.

Workmen start at the ceiling and work down, vacuuming every surface, doing the floor last. Once the HEPA vacuuming is done, every surface is washed with a lead-binding solution. HUD interim guidelines, issued in 1990, call for the use of detergents with high phosphate content, typically 5 percent Tri-Sodium Phosphate (TSP). (See "Do the Easy Things First," pp. 22–23.) The problem is that phosphates are harmful to the environment, and are regulated or banned in 35 states. A new product may resolve the problem. LEDIZOLV, developed and manufactured by Hin-Cor Industries of Beaufort, South Carolina (1-803-522-3066), has been shown to bind five times as much lead as TSP and is totally phosphate free. The EPA is in the process of designing a study to test the effectiveness of LEDIZOLV (and other products), and Hin-Cor is trying to establish national hardware store distribution of its product. If you have the option, use a phosphate substitute.

After everything has dried, the whole cycle—HEPA vacuuming followed by phosphate washdown—is repeated. Finally, because particles of lead dust can remain airborne for a considerable length of time, the cycle is repeated after the home has been repainted.

Homeowners without access to a HEPAvac can improve their cleanup of lead-paint dust by washing with a lead-binding detergent solution and then vacuuming with a wet-and-dry vacuum cleaner while the surfaces remain wet. Never dry-vacuum lead-paint chips or dust with anything but a HEPAvac.

TAX DEDUCTIONS FOR ABATEMENT

The only good news in all this is that abatement work is tax deductible, either as a medical expense or as a capital improvement. Internal Revenue Service (IRS) Publication 502, "Medical and Dental Expenses," states:

> You can include in medical expenses the cost of removing lead-based paints from surfaces in your home to prevent a child who has or has had lead poisoning from eating the paint. These surfaces must be in poor repair (peeling or cracking) or within the child's reach. The cost of repainting the scraped area is not a medical expense.
>
> If, instead of removing the paint, you cover the area with wallboard or paneling, treat these items as capital expenses. See capital expenses, earlier. Do not include the cost of painting the wallboard as a medical expense.

This is definitely a time to confer with a tax specialist. IRS guidance is minimal and vague, and you are potentially talking about a lot of money. Note that a child living in the house or apartment must have been diagnosed as lead poisoned before the lead-paint removal can be considered a deductible medical expense.

BEFORE YOU REPAINT . . .

The final step in any abatement project—before you repaint, before it's safe for children to reenter the area—is what's called clearance testing, a visual inspection to make sure all lead paint has been abated in one way or another, coupled with a dust-sample test. Dust samples are usually taken from the floor next to the abated surfaces and from windowsills and window wells. They may also be taken from outside the work area to ensure that contamination did not spread. Dust-sample testing should be done by someone other than the abatement contractor.

The EPA has established new standards for dust testing. They are 11 $\mu g/ft^2$ (micrograms of lead per square foot) for floors, 500 $\mu g/ft^2$ for windowsills, and 800 $\mu g/ft^2$ for window wells. Areas that test below these levels are considered acceptable for human occupancy. Your local health department can tell you if more stringent levels have been established where you live.

Even after interior lead paint has been successfully abated, you should continue to wash your home occasionally with a lead-binding solution to remove any ambient lead dust that may have blown or been tracked in from outdoors.

PRECAUTIONS TO TAKE WITH SMALL PROJECTS

Any project, however small, that disturbs lead paint increases the risk that your child will be exposed to lead. You can minimize that risk by taking certain precautions:

- Keep children out of the work area, preferably out of the home, until work—including cleanup—is done.
- Never power-sand, dry-sand, or dry-scrape lead paint.
- Carefully mask the area. Tape down a disposable drop cloth to catch any chips or plaster that may fall. Cover any carpeting or upholstered furniture that can't be moved out of the room.
- Close off the room. Close the window so there is no draft to spread contamination. Tape plastic over any heat vents, especially cold-air intakes.
- Have plastic bags on hand to hold any debris that's being removed. Save one for your clothes—they should be washed separately—when the job is done.
- Wet the paint area with a spray bottle of phosphate-detergent solution before disturbing the paint. Keep spraying as you work to keep dust from flying.
- Knicks and chips in otherwise solid lead-based paint should be wet-sanded and touched up before a toddler starts picking at the edges and lifting small chips and dust.
- Wipe every surface and mop the floor with the phosphate or other lead-binding detergent solution when the job is done.
- It's best, if possible, to pass bags of debris out a window rather than carrying them through your home.
- Be careful not to track dust and debris into other rooms. Change clothes before you leave the room. Make sure your hair (including your beard) doesn't carry a load of dust out of the work area.
- You may want to rent a HEPAvac if you feel the above precautions didn't capture and contain all possible dust and debris.

RESEARCH IN LEAD-PAINT ABATEMENT

Dr. Mark Farfel has been studying lead-paint abatement in Baltimore since the days when landlords would hire torchmen—untrained day-laborers—off the streets to burn paint off tenement woodwork. That was nearly two decades ago; Baltimore was one of the first cities in the nation to require lead-paint abatement where a child became lead poisoned.

The original Baltimore law was based on the premise that children became lead poisoned by eating lead paint. Landlords had to remove lead paint to a height of four feet above the floor. They could sand, scrape, or burn the paint off, hence the proliferation of torchmen.

The abatement was a failure. Dr. Farfel's studies showed that children who were chelated and returned to housing units abated by torching and sanding were inevitably rehospitalized with a second case of lead poisoning. Dr. Farfel, who is an assistant professor at Johns Hopkins University, conducted field studies tracking lead-dust levels before and after abatement.

"Lead-dust levels were higher after abatement than they were before," he says, "and they were still higher six to nine months later."

It took ten more years, but Dr. Farfel's findings finally brought about change in Baltimore's law. In 1987, burning and sanding were prohibited, the four-foot limit was lifted, and postabatement cleanup and testing were required. Baltimore's law became Maryland law a year later and eventually became the basis for the HUD document setting national lead abatement standards.

Today, Dr. Farfel is project director for a Kennedy Krieger Institute study that is looking for ways to cut the cost of abating lead paint without putting children at risk. Three different levels of repair and maintenance—estimated to cost $1,600, $3,500, and $7,000 respectively for a typical 1,200-square-foot two-story row house—are being compared to both new and previously abated dwellings to determine just how much abatement is needed to protect the health of our children.

It's important research; too many people—and too many cities and states—have been so intimidated by the potential cost of lead abatement that they are doing nothing. The hazard of lead paint will not go away by itself.

5

SOIL

A child will eat a peck of dirt before he dies.

— *Grandma Stapleton*

WHEN THE EPA TESTS an industrial waste site and finds lead levels of 1,000 ppm in the ground, the soil is considered toxic, and the site qualifies for remedial action under the Superfund program. Cleanup standards for residential sites are 400 ppm. When Anne Sheehan tested her backyard, she found lead levels as high as 5,000 ppm. "We couldn't even have the dirt hauled away," she says. "It's considered hazardous waste."

The Sheehans are not alone. Yards in Staten Island, New York, have been tested at 1,000 to 4,000 ppm lead; they are downwind from a lead smelting facility in nearby New Jersey. Houses with front yards on busy roadways typically have soil-lead levels up to 2,000 ppm; the roadside lead pollution is residual contamination left over from the days of leaded gasoline. Garden soil in the center of Baltimore, Maryland, tested as high as 10,000 ppm, reflecting contamination from a combination of urban sources. Lead doesn't biodegrade or decay; it remains in the soil forever. Or until a child eats it.

My grandmother may have exaggerated the amount, but kids do eat dirt. A few, pica children, eat it by the handful. The rest ingest sprinkles of dirt coincidentally as they run in from playing in the yard and grab a cookie or carrot in grubby little hands. Even when they're not eating, children frequently have their hands in their mouths during play activity. All of this is normal and quite benign, unless your yard happens to have contaminated soil. Unfortunately, for all too many of us, that's the case. Dr. Tom Spitler of the EPA regional office in Boston estimates most kids ingest 50–100 mg of dirt a day; if that dirt contains even 1,000 ppm lead, the child will consume enough lead to suffer low-level lead poisoning.

CONTAMINATION FROM LEAD PAINT

The greatest contributor to lead contamination of yard soil is paint. How many times have you seen people scraping their gutters or porches or having their exterior sanded without even so much as a drop cloth on the ground? How many times has this happened to your house? And not just while you lived there, but going back through previous owners, because the lead carried in paint chips never goes away. Every chip and particle of lead paint that falls to the ground when a house is prepped for repainting raises the level of lead contamination.

Even if your house was never scraped or sanded, if it's old enough to have been coated with lead paint (pre-1980, possible; pre-1960, likely; pre-1940, almost certainly), the normal action of rain and snow has washed lead chalk into your yard. A survey in New Haven, Connecticut, found the lead levels in soil close to homes built around 1975 averaged less than 150 ppm, whereas lead levels in soil close to homes built before 1940 were eight times as high.

Lead-paint contamination of soil isn't limited to the perimeter of houses; you'll find it near out-buildings, including garages and barns, under painted fences, and even where rusting vehicles or farm equipment may have stood. City dwellers may find their property being contaminated with lead paint coming from overhead bridges and highways.

If your child has a sandbox, make sure it's not close to any source of lead-based paint. Move it away from the foundation. Don't store it under a porch painted with lead-based paint. If your neighborhood is filled with older homes having lead paint, keep the sandbox covered. If you or a neighbor has done any exterior work since the sandbox was last filled, change the sand. Health officials say one of the most commonly overlooked sources of childhood lead exposure is the innocent sandbox.

Most soil-lead contamination remains very close to the surface.

Lead is actually immobilized by the organic components of soil, and unless your ground has been turned or worked by gardening, the lead that has come off your house is still sitting in the top inch or two of earth.

There's no mystery where the lead in Anne and Kevin Sheehan's yard came from. The exterior of their house was in bad shape when they bought it; paint was peeling from the porch, cracked and alligatored on the clapboard siding. The contract on their fix-it-up FHA mortgage required them to repaint, after first removing all loose paint. The Sheehans scraped what they could and power-sanded the rest. By the time they were done, their yard looked as if there had been an out-of-season snowstorm.

And then 30-month-old Kate was discovered to be lead poisoned. The Sheehans started testing for lead and quickly realized that the cloud of white paint that blew from their house had carried with it a deadly precipitate. Every spot they tested in their yard exceeded the EPA's 500 ppm threshold for residential soil.* Anne and Kevin had created a hazardous waste site in their own backyard, so toxic it had to be declared off-limits to their three children.

The EPA doesn't clean individual yards, but the Sheehans decided to adapt a standard Superfund remedy: They capped their backyard, burying the lead contamination beneath a six-inch layer of clay and soil. It took five dump-truck loads—each containing more than 20 tons of dirt—just to cover behind their home. Close to the house, where the contamination was highest, Kevin laid a brick patio to put yet another layer of protection between the children and the lead. State health officials were involved because of the lead poisoning, and they required that the cap material be tested for lead before it was brought on site. The dirt, which came from a supermarket construction site, tested okay, but the first batch of brick, donated by a neighbor who was tearing down a chimney, had to be rejected; it too was contaminated with lead paint.

CONTAMINATION FROM AUTOMOBILE EXHAUST

The second major source of lead contamination in soil came from automobile exhaust. Although lead emissions from car engines are no

*The EPA is currently considering lowering this threshold to 400 ppm.

longer a significant source of lead pollution—the EPA calls the reduction of airborne lead pollution one of its greatest success stories— ATSDR estimates that four to five million tons of pre-1986 auto-exhaust lead is still in the dust and soil along our streets and highways. Studies found levels of soil-lead in frontyards to be two to three times higher than levels in backyards. Soil-lead levels are higher close to streets and roadways, and they are highest, up to 10,000 ppm, close to heavily traveled and congested roads having stop-and-go traffic. This legacy of auto-exhaust lead contamination is of greater concern in urban areas than in rural; lead levels are higher in cities because of greater traffic volume and since backyards are smaller, kids tend to play out front, where soil-lead levels are highest.

CONTAMINATION NEAR ELEVATED STEEL STRUCTURES

People who live near or under highway bridges got a double dose of lead contamination. Not only did the lead-contaminated exhaust from passing vehicles blow down on homes and yards, but as the bridges gradually rust, they rain flakes of industrial exterior-grade lead paint, which can be as much as 90 percent lead, on the property below. This is true of any elevated steel structure, including railway bridges and electrical transmission towers. The shower of contamination becomes a deluge when workers have to sandblast the old paint from the old ironwork.

A classic study published in the *New England Journal of Medicine* in 1982 focused on the Mystic River Bridge, connecting Boston's Charlestown section with Chelsea, Massachusetts. The high suspension bridge passes over densely populated sections of the city, and it was found to be shedding great flakes of lead paint. Soil samples in yards below ranged from 1,300 to 4,800 ppm, and a pediatric survey of children living under the bridge in Chelsea found that 49 percent of them had blood-lead levels above 30 μg/dl, which was the CDC action level at the time (it's now 10 μg/dl).

In 1979, the Massachusetts Port Authority, owner of the bridge, decided to remove lead-based paint from sections of the bridge that passed over housing; abrasive blasting was begun in suspended enclosures sealed to the bridge with canvas shrouds. The lead-paint chips and used grit were carried to containers on the ground in large hoses.

There were, however, leaks in the hoses and from the enclosures.

Spent sand containing paint chips accumulated on the homes and in the yards beneath the workmen. The state Department of Environmental Quality tested the air near the work and found lead levels almost nine times the EPA standards. Levels of lead in the sand/paint mix that collected under the bridge ranged as high as 12,900 ppm.

Massachusetts officials, including the Port Authority, worked with federal health experts to improve lead containment, and the measures taken were fully discussed in the *Journal* article. Yet 10 years later, residents of Brooklyn, New York's Williamsburg section found themselves being showered with grit and lead paint from sandblasting operations on the Williamsburg Bridge that hovered over their homes.

TESTING AND ABATING LEAD IN SOIL

Any home survey that's looking for possible sources of lead contamination must at least consider soil. The older your home and the homes and buildings around it, the closer you are to traffic, or to overhead steel structures or to a lead-based industry (which we'll discuss later in this chapter), the greater the risk that lead has contaminated your soil. If your home is in a brand-new subdivision carved out of virgin farmland, chances are pretty good there's no lead in the soil, but I would still test it. On the farm I grew up on, now home to several houses, there are hot spots of lead contamination where no one would suspect—one at the edge of a pasture, where pieces of derelict machinery sat to rust, shedding their load of red lead paint; another in a remote field, where a hay shed burned one night, leaving a pile of lead-contaminated ash.

Testing soil for lead is cheap and simple. State Agricultural Extension Services in a number of states (Massachusetts, Minnesota, New York, Pennsylvania, Wisconsin, and the District of Columbia) provide inexpensive soil-lead tests. If your state's Cooperative Extension Service doesn't offer soil testing, you may turn to the University of the District of Columbia for help. UDC is a land-grant institution in the nation's capital, and Environmental Sciences Professor James R. Preer uses soil testing as a teaching tool. He's agreed to accept soil testing requests from anywhere in the United States. UDC will send you an instruction sheet and a bag to mail back your soil sample. Students will test your soil for lead, cadmium, copper, zinc, iron, and nickel as well as for pH. Cost, including a sheet explaining the results, is $10.

Write:

Agricultural Experiment Station
University of the District of Columbia
4200 Connecticut Avenue NW
Washington, DC 20008

Your local public health officials should also be able to recommend commercial labs that will test soil, or you may call your state lead resource listed in appendix D. If a large number of samples need to be tested, portable XRF testing equipment (see chapter 3) may also be used.

If you find that your soil is contaminated, you'll need to take steps to eliminate it as a source of lead poisoning. Lead does not naturally work its way down through soil, so if the area of contamination is limited, it may make sense to remove the top one or two inches of dirt and replace it with new topsoil. Wet the soil down as you remove it to keep lead dust from spreading. Either the contaminated soil should be bagged for inclusion with municipal trash, or it should be buried on site. Dig a hole large and deep enough to hold both the leaded soil and a 12-inch cap of clean topsoil. If possible, locate this buried soil where it will not be later disturbed, and where you can plant grass or some other ground cover. Don't dig up lead-contaminated soil only to dump it where it can blow about or erode to expose someone else at a later date.

The EPA recently completed a series of tests to determine the effectiveness of efforts to remove lead contamination in urban soil. Tests were run in Boston, Baltimore, and Cincinnati; a different set of circumstances was studied in each city, but they covered soil abatement, dust removal, and paint stabilization. Soil abatement involved excavation and removal. Dust removal entailed street and hand sweeping. Paint stabilization meant the removal of chipping and peeling paint that might recontaminate the soil that had been cleaned up. Children's blood-lead levels were monitored before and after removal of contaminated soil and dust.

The study found that lead moves freely throughout a child's environment. Lead in paint becomes lead in soil; lead in soil becomes lead in street or playground dust; lead in street dust becomes lead in house dust. Digging up and removing contaminated soil did in fact lower the level of lead in children's blood. But the cost was astronomical. Dr. Michael Weitzman of the University of Rochester School of Medicine and Dentistry participated in the project and wrote about its findings in the *Journal of the American Medical Association*. The modest reduction in blood-lead levels was "not enough," he says, "to justify digging up significant portions of inner cities throughout the United States." Weitzman says the soil sampling, testing, removal, and replacement cost nearly $10,000 per property. That seems incredibly high given the small area of earth removed—ATSDR, in its 1987 "Report to Congress," estimated the cost of removing the top three inches of soil in a typical Boston yard to be $1,357 including disposal in a lined landfill—but compared to the cost of abating lead paint in an inner-city housing unit, which has far greater impact on the reduction of childhood lead poisoning, soil removal on any significant scale—as national policy as opposed to individual action—seems neither practical nor economical.

Capping is often the simplest and most effective way for the homeowner to deal with lead-contaminated soil. Planting a lawn will often be enough to protect small children by isolating lead-laden dirt. Dr. Weitzman suggests that simply adding several inches of clean topsoil would be far less expensive and also far less intrusive than excavation. Planting shrubs around the foundation and adding a heavy layer of mulch will also create a barrier. However, you'll need to keep an eye on kids and pets. Shrubs and hedges may say "Keep out!" to adults, but they are often an inviting hiding place for children at play. Dogs like to sleep in the shade under foundation plantings—some like to dig and sleep—and they will carry a load of contaminated dust into the house in their fur. The Sheehan's solution of covering the area of worst contamination with a patio combines utility and beauty while offering the greatest protection against lead exposure.

TO BEET OR NOT TO BEET

No discussion of lead contamination in soil would be complete without talking about gardening. Who doesn't relish home-grown veggies? From a tomato plant in a fire-escape flower pot to the neatly tended rows of a farm garden, food you grow yourself just seems so much better. It's fresher. Fewer people have handled it. You can control the use of pesticides. But if there is lead lurking in the soil around your home, there is the danger that backyard veggies will either absorb the lead or carry lead-laden soil into your house. Depending on where and how they're grown, home-grown vegetables may contain considerably more lead than commercial produce at the neighborhood grocery.

While eating vegetables grown in lead-contaminated soil will add to your family's lead intake, and is certainly a risk, by far the greater risk, especially to small children, is the dirt itself. It's carried into the house on the vegetables and on your hands, shoes, and clothing. Crawling infants who are years away from eating spinach and beets will carry the dirt to their mouths through normal hand-to-mouth activity. The danger from soil carried into the home is five to ten times that posed by the worst class of vegetables.

You should avoid planting:

■ In soil contaminated with flaking or scraped exterior paint; such as soil found in garden plots bordering the house, garage, barn, or other buildings.

■ In soil heavily exposed in the past to automobile exhaust; such as soil found in street-level urban gardens or near rural highways.

■ In soil exposed to pollution (including air pollution) from the factory of a lead-based industry such as a smelter, battery manufacturer, or radiator repair shop.

People in the country tend to grow their vegetables in real gardens, patches ranging from quilt size up to, depending on who's weeding, a small field. But suburbanites and city people, confined to smaller lots, often intermix vegetables with flowers in border gardens. If these border gardens are up against the house or garage, or even an old painted fence, their soil may be laced with lead from deteriorated paint. Every shard of peeling paint that breaks or is scraped off falls to the ground below. It joins the lead chalk that has been washed into the soil by rainwater. These soils have been found to be contaminated with lead levels in excess of 10,000 ppm. You may also find pockets of high-level lead pollution stemming from other industrial or professional sources. A previous owner or neighbor may have been a painter who cleaned his brushes behind the garage, or a potter whose glaze or paints spilled onto the soil. Before you plant a garden, test the soil.

The laudable move to convert vacant city lots into urban gardens has to contend with the likelihood that existing soil is contaminated with lead. If the lot has been vacant for years, it may be contaminated with lead from auto exhaust (especially true of corner lots near stop signs and traffic lights). If it is newly vacant, the result of tearing an old building down, the soil may be heavy with lead-paint contamination. The soil on urban lots is generally poor growing soil anyway, and the best bet there may be to truck in new topsoil.

As to what produce to grow, agronomist Rufus Chaney, with the U.S. Department of Agriculture's Environmental Chemistry Lab, says lead accumulates first in the plant's stem and leaves, then in its roots, and finally, a distant third, in its flowers and fruit. This means that leafy vegetables such as lettuce, spinach, and cabbage and root vegetables like potatoes, carrots, and onions will carry much higher levels of lead than tomatoes, cucumbers, beans, and corn.

One of the first things my mother gave me to grow was radish seed. I'll never understand why . . . I don't know many kids who like to eat radishes . . . but that seems to be a gardening tradition. If you're intent on continuing this tradition, and there's lead in your soil, have your child grow her radishes in a flowerpot or potting tray with new soil.

If the only plot available for gardening shows some lead, but not so much that gardening must be ruled out, there are some things you can do to lessen the amount of lead your plants will take up. Agronomist Chaney recommends the following steps:

- Keep the soil pH level above 6.5. Garden centers sell inexpensive kits that measure pH. To raise the level, add limestone. Fifty pounds per 1,000 square feet will raise the pH one point (1.0).
- Add phosphates. Phosphate is the middle number of the

SOIL LEAD LEVELS AND GARDEN VEGETABLES

LEVEL	ACTION
50–500 ppm	Rinse dirt off vegetables and your hands and knees while outdoors, wash the vegetables.
500–1,000 ppm	Above, plus limit consumption of leafy and root vegetables.
1,000–3,000 ppm	Above, except do not grow or eat leafy or root vegetables.
3,000-plus ppm	Do not garden (either vegetables or flowers) in this soil. Replace it, or move the garden.

three-number series you see on bags of fertilizer. Thus 5-10-10 fertilizer is 10 percent phosphate.

■ Add organic matter. Manure, peat moss, mulch, and compost will all help, but note that both organic matter and fertilizers will lower the soil's pH. Fifty pounds of peat moss per 1,000 square feet of garden will help bind lead, but it will also *drop* the pH one point. Add lime too.

Without getting into the chemistry of all this, the net result is these measures make it more difficult for the plant to pull the lead out of the soil. They don't, however, keep your little person from eating the soil, so keep the garden dirt out of the house (and isn't that what your mother always told you anyway?).

Scientists are studying the effects of using sludge compost in vegetable gardens. Sludge, which is a by-product of the treatment of sewage, is an excellent fertilizer. However, waste treatment does not remove heavy metals, and the use of sludge compost has been shown to increase the level of lead in soil. Yet the short-term use of sludge compost, applied at typical rates, has not been shown to increase lead levels in vegetables raised in the soil. The long-term effects are not known. I would avoid the use of sludge compost in any soil whose lead content is already questionable.

INDUSTRIAL HAZARDS

Soil contamination from lead paint and automobile exhaust is a threat all of us have to deal with to one degree or another. Some communities, however, face far greater risk; they were—or still are—home to some offshoot of the lead industry. Smelters, battery factories, automobile radiator shops, and even some recycling facilities generate lead pollution. People living near active factories, with today's pollution controls, may be at less risk than people living near abandoned facilities, which spewed lead contamination with gay abandon in the days before environmental controls were put in place. The EPA says total lead emissions have dropped from 20,100 tons in 1985, when leaded gas was still being sold, to 5,200 tons in 1992. EPA's latest report on air quality identifies areas that exceed the current standards for airborne lead pollution. These high levels were all the result of pollution from industrial sources.

CITY/AREA	1990 POPULATION	AIR-LEAD LEVEL
Birmingham, Ala.	908,000	1.15
Cleveland, Ohio	1,831,000	37.40
Columbus, Ga./Ala.	243,000	1.46
Dallas-Ft. Worth, Tex.	2,553,000	0.91
Dent, Mo.	1,000	*
Douglas, Nebr.	<1,000	*
Indianapolis, Ind.	1,250,000	1.53
Lewis & Clark, Mont.	2,000	
Liberty-Arcadia, Mo.	6,000	*
Memphis, Tenn./Ark./Miss.	982,000	1.84
Minneapolis-St. Paul, Minn./Wis.	2,464,000	0.89
Nashville, Tenn.	985,000	0.83
Omaha, Nebr./Iowa	618,000	4.51
Philadelphia, Pa./N.J.	4,857,000	17.60
St. Louis, Mo./Ill.	2,444,000	11.80

*Levels for non-Metropolitan Statistical Area villages were not listed.

Source: EPA *National Air Quality And Emissions Trends Report,* 1992.

In 1991, the EPA announced a Multi-Media Lead Strategy designed to reduce lead levels at a total of 31 industrial sources, mostly lead smelters, through a combination of enforcement and negotiation with the industries involved.

Smelters have historically been the worst offenders. They heat either ore or scrap metal to melt and separate out metals, and soil tests near smelters have measured lead contamination as high as 100,000 ppm. The plume of pollution from a smelter can travel for miles through either air or groundwater (groundwater is water that pools or flows underground).

ATSDR recently conducted a health study at the site of the Zinc Corporation of America in Bartlesville, Oklahoma. Smelting operations began there in 1907, and air emissions were essentially uncontrolled until 1976. Blood-lead levels of local children in a late 1970s survey *averaged* 28 µg/dl, and almost 40 percent of the children had blood-lead levels above 30 µg/dl, which was the CDC threshold at the time.

The new survey tested air and soil in a 36-square-mile area around the smelter, which is still active. Areas of lead contamination were identified, and health officials conducted a new study of blood-lead levels. More than 10 percent of the children in the target area tested above the current CDC threshold of 10 μg/dl; there were no children above that level in a control group. According to ATSDR, there was a significant relationship between elevated blood-lead levels and distance from the old smelter. The EPA has spent $2.5 million removing lead-contaminated soil from 30 so-called high-access sites, meaning schools, playgrounds, and day-care facilities. The agency is now starting clean-up work in residential areas where the lead concentration is above 1,500 ppm. More than eight square miles will eventually have to be cleaned up.

The prevalence of lead contamination is underscored by the results of similar ATSDR public health assessments. ATSDR is called in to evaluate suspect sites to determine the risk to people's health. In 1992, the most recent year for which figures are available, 79 percent of the sites that ATSDR found to be public health hazards contained lead contamination. The lead at most of these was in the soil or groundwater. The most common recommendations were to fence-in the property to keep people, especially children, from having contact with the lead and to prohibit the drilling of wells that could tap the polluted water supply.

Typical was the situation at the Waite Park Wells Superfund site in Waite Park, Minnesota. Burlington Northern repaired and rebuilt railroad cars at the site. As part of refurbishing the old cars, paint was sandblasted off them, and the paint-laden sand was piled on an open lot directly across the street from an elementary school. Lead levels in the sand were over 6,000 ppm, and in the soil under the sand, levels reached a staggering 120,000 ppm. As a result of EPA action, the contamination has been covered with heavy plastic to keep it from being blown about, and the site has been fenced to keep the schoolchildren from playing in the sand.

Not all contamination from smelters traveled through the air. A lead recycling smelter in Granite City, Illinois, which recovered lead from old car batteries, solved its trash disposal problem years ago by offering crushed battery casings to anyone who would haul them away. Local residents lined up to truck it off. The hard rubber casings made excellent fill, especially good in driveways, and the nearby town of Venice used it to pave municipal alleys. A health study of the area found that one out of every six children between the ages of six months and six years has elevated blood-lead levels, and the EPA is now involved in a seven-year, $30-million project to remove lead contamination from some 55 blocks of Granite City and three other localities.

The town of Stratford, Connecticut, faces a similar problem, though from a different source. ATSDR declared in 1993 that an urgent public health threat exists in the town because of widespread lead, asbestos, and PCB contamination, including the ball fields at an intermediate school. For almost 70 years, a company that manufactured brake pads dumped its industrial sludge in waste pits. Every so often, the pits would be drained, and the sludge mixed with dirt. The dirt/sludge mix, loaded with contaminants, was then trucked off by anyone, including the town, who needed fill to reclaim the swampy land that proliferated along the Stratford River.

There is a mystery in all of this. It's clear that soil-borne lead contributes to lead poisoning—the number of childhood lead-poisoning cases peaks during summer months, when children are playing more outdoors and when outdoor activity brings lead-laced soil into the house. What's not clear is why some soil-lead contamination contributes more to blood-lead levels than others. Some Superfund sites, some communities even, register enormous levels of lead contamination, yet the potential risk is not necessarily reflected in people's blood-lead levels. Different studies have determined wide-ranging differences in the relationship between soil-lead levels and children's blood-lead levels. Theories abound, based on such variables as the size of the lead particles or chemical form of the lead, which would both affect the rate at which the body absorbs lead, and the child's behavior patterns, including amount of hand-to-mouth activity, access to the soil, or the presence of ground cover. In the meantime, since we don't understand the relationship, prudence dictates that we do everything practical to either eliminate soil-lead contamination or put some barrier between it and our children.

WASTE DISPOSAL AND LEAD

There's growing concern today over the trend toward the incineration of municipal garbage. You probably know that if you toss an old car battery in the trash, you're throwing out a big lump of lead, but many small batteries contain lead too. So does the ink on consumer packaging and colored newsprint. And every time you throw out an old stereo or radio, loaded with solder, or an old door, covered with layers of lead paint, you add another source of lead to the waste stream. The stream of municipal waste flows to the incinerator to be burned, but lead doesn't burn, and without proper controls, municipal incinerators may become major new sources of airborne lead pollution. The American Public Health Association estimates that more than one million pounds of lead particles are emitted into the air by incinerators every year.

The most efficient way to prevent this is to keep lead from getting into the waste stream. Several states have banned the incineration of lead-acid batteries; instead they require separate collection and recycling. New York has gone farther, strictly limiting the amount of lead in consumer packaging. This action will have the beneficial side effect of eliminating another potential contributor to childhood lead poisoning, because lead-foil caps on wine bottles and lead pigments in the inks on food packages will be forced out of the home.

While recycling is reducing the number of lead-acid batteries that go into the trash, the computer industry is adding a new source of waste lead. When you dump an old TV set or computer monitor, you're adding a large source of lead to your municipal garbage, for the glass in the cathode-ray-tube (CRT) viewing screens of TVs and computer monitors contains a high percent of lead in order to protect viewers from harmful radiation. A university study estimates that 10 million computers are being discarded every year. CRTs account for more than a quarter of the total lead disposed in municipal waste, 52,000 tons in 1986! While the EPA is considering declaring CRTs hazardous waste to better control their disposition, a CRT recycling industry is evolving, and one company, Environcycle, reports it has successfully processed more than 1.5 million pounds of leaded CRT glass, much of it to be made into new CRTs.

Amendments to the Clean Air Act passed in 1990 required the EPA to set standards for the amount of lead allowed out of the smokestack of a solid waste incinerator. The EPA, which believes that mechanical devices like scrubbers, required to remove other smokestack pollutants, catch whatever lead emissions may be there, missed the deadline for setting lead emission standards, and was sued by the Natural Resources Defense Council (NRDC). The standards are now due, under court order, by the end of 1994.

A potentially more significant piece of legislation, the Lead Exposure Reduction Act, remains stalled on Capitol Hill. If passed, this broad act would significantly reduce the amount of lead introduced into both our lives and our environment (see chapter 11) and would mean that less lead will make its way into the waste stream.

6

LEAD AND DRINKING WATER

Plumbing, from Latin plumbum, *lead.*
Plumber, from Latin plumbārius, *lead*
worker.

—*American Heritage Dictionary*

MARGARET BENNET* had lusty lungs when she was an infant. Each morning, when she woke up hungry, her crying sent her parents scurrying downstairs to the kitchen, where they ran some hot water and made her a bottle of formula. Her family was shocked when a routine blood-lead screen showed that Margaret was being lead poisoned.

Tom Spitler wasn't. According to Spitler, the EPA's regional lead expert, "They did everything wrong. They used hot instead of cold water. They didn't let the water run. They just didn't know." When Spitler tested a sample of the water Margaret's parents were using to make her formula, he found it contained over 500 ppb lead (the EPA standard is 15 ppb). On his recommendation, the family changed to bottled water for Margaret's formula and juices, and her blood-lead levels quickly came back down.

Lead in our drinking water is rarely the only cause of lead poisoning, but it's often a contributing factor, especially for infants and toddlers. The concentration of lead in the body is cumulative, and drinking water can add significantly to the total amount of lead a person is exposed to. The EPA estimates that 10 to 20 percent of the average

*In order to protect individual's privacy, real name has been changed.

person's daily lead intake comes from drinking water. The body absorbs lead in drinking water more readily than lead in food: Adults absorb 35 to 50 percent of the lead they drink; the figure is higher for children.

Babies and toddlers drink a lot of water. We make their formula with it. We cut their fruit juice with it. We make their cereal with it. And every time we mix in a little water, we're mixing in a dose of lead. Lead in water may account for as much as 50 percent of a small child's total lead intake.

Don't think that boiling the water will make it safe from lead. Boiling will kill germs, but you can't "kill" lead. In fact, letting water boil actually increases the concentration of lead. Babies have been poisoned when hot tap water was boiled to make their formula. Take note: *Until you have tested your water and checked your plumbing system, the safest thing to do is to use bottled water for your infant or toddler.*

But do test your water. Testing is the only way to know how much lead is in your drinking water. Every home has a different level of lead in its drinking water, and *every faucet* will deliver a different level of lead.

There's a very good chance that you do *not* have a lead problem. In fact, the nation's leading water-lead research program, at the University of North Carolina-Ashville, has tested the water from more than 60,000 homes. It found that 83 percent of the homes tested had no problem with lead. Another 15 percent could solve their problem simply by running the water briefly before using it. Depending on the results, a water-lead test will either give you peace of mind or prompt you to take preventive action.

AN AGE-OLD PROBLEM

It's maddening that we should even be concerned with water as a source of lead. This is not a new problem. Drinking water has been poisoned with lead at least since the time of the Roman Empire. At the same time Rome's water commissioner was writing about the city's elaborate lead-pipe water system, the scholar Pliny was describing classic symptoms of lead poisoning among the slaves working Roman lead mines. Sixteen centuries later, the Massachusetts Bay Colony banned the use of lead in stills because local rum was poisoning people. In 1845, a report on Boston's water supplies concluded that, "considering the deadly nature of lead poison, . . . it is certainly [in] the cause of safety to avoid . . . the use of lead pipe for carrying water which is to be used for drinking." Yet the city of Boston permitted lead water lines for another century, and Chicago's building code called for lead service lines until 1986.

Lead supply lines are still around. Not only in Rome and Boston and Chicago but in New York and Baltimore and countless other cities and towns. We found one coming into our house. It pokes through the foundation wall, sagging and curving like an unsupported snake. It's been painted white, along with the basement walls, but when I scraped at it with a knife, the soft metal cut, revealing a telltale patch of shiny silver metal.

Lead would appear to be a natural choice for plumbing. It's cheap and plentiful; durable, soft, and easily malleable. Best of all, it doesn't rust. Lead has been used not only to deliver water but to line everything from cisterns to the tanks in water coolers. The use of solid lead in water supply systems was allowed in the United States right up to 1986, when the Safe Drinking Water Act was amended.

The problem is that water will slowly extract lead from the solid metal and carry it to your faucet and, ultimately, into your body. Sometimes the faucet itself is the source of the lead. The following are all potential sources of contamination:

- Lead service lines
- Lead connectors
- Lead pipes
- Lead tank lining
- Copper pipe connected with lead solder
- Brass or bronze faucets
- Chrome-plated faucets

The extraction process is called *leaching*. You use the process everyday to make coffee. When hot water is passed over ground coffee beans, it extracts the chemicals that convert the water into America's favorite morning brew. Just as hot water makes stronger coffee than cold water, hot water leaches lead at a faster rate than cold. Lead-leaching rates are affected by a number of factors, including heat, and they can act in concert to quickly concoct a deadly brew.

LEAD LEACHING FROM FAUCETS

How often have you gotten up early in the morning and run a half-glass of water to take a pill? Or to give to your toddler? That shiny silver faucet in your bathroom or kitchen is a major source of lead. It's made of brass—the silver is actually a thin plating of chrome—and brass is an alloy containing lead.

Faucets are of special concern as a lead source since water sits in them for prolonged periods. When you go into the kitchen first thing to draw water for coffee, you're running water that has had all night to suck lead out of the kitchen faucet's brass.

How much lead does that "first draw" of water contain? The same law (1986) that banned lead pipes also limited the lead content of brass plumbing fixtures to eight percent but the state of California wanted to know what this translated to at the tap. The state turned to the Environmental Quality Institute (EQI) at the University of North Carolina-Ashville, the nation's largest research center devoted to the study of lead in drinking water. Director Richard P. Maas tested 19 brands of faucets for lead leaching. He found that on the average, 30 percent of the lead in "first draw" water came from the brass in the faucet. But the results showed a huge disparity. California's deputy attorney general, Edward Weil, learned that when it comes to leaching lead, not all brass faucets are created equal. The California tests show that the manufacturing process can make a big difference in how much of that lead can be leached from a given faucet.

"Don't be fooled by shiny kitchen faucets," warns Weil. "You can't tell by looking. Chrome plating covers up the sandcast brass." Price is no gauge either. The California tests found inexpensive faucets that leached only low levels of lead, and expensive faucets that were sandcast brass. Brand-name recognition doesn't mean anything either; Price-Pfister, which sells more faucets in California than any other company, had the second-highest levels of lead leaching.

There are three different ways to make a brass faucet. *Fabrication* essentially means the faucet is carved out of solid brass. In *permanent mold casting,* molten brass is poured—cast—into a reusable mold. In *sandcasting,* the molten brass is poured into a sand mold that is later broken to remove the faucet. For reasons too technical to get into here, the sandcasting process results in more of the brass alloy's lead content migrating to the surface as the metal cools. Since your water does its leaching at the metal surface, sandcast faucets leach at a far higher rate than the others.

How much higher? After taking into account the amount of water each faucet contained, Professor Maas was able to provide comparative values for the various faucets. The best faucets, in terms of leaching, introduced less than 4.5 µg of lead into the water. The worst, from

Chicago and Price-Pfister, both very popular brands, loaded the water with 124.8 and 76.8 μg of lead respectively. Remember that for infants and toddlers, 60 μg of lead translates into a blood-lead level of 10 μg/dl, the CDC action level.

California sued the faucet manufacturers under its Proposition 65, requiring the companies to attach warning labels to their products. Professor Maas testified before the California State Superior Court: "To put this in practical terms, a typical faucet has a volume of between 30 and 150 milliliters (1 to 5 ounces). A consumer drinking tap water over the course of a day will ingest the full amount of lead indicated in Exhibit C [124.8 micrograms, for instance], or an amount close to this, *each time that he or she drinks a glass of water when the faucet has been turned off for 2 hours or more*" (emphasis mine).

Or each time you make a baby's bottle. Buried in the EQI research is a startling finding that challenges the conventional wisdom on how to flush lead out of your pipes. You're presently advised to flush your system in the morning by running water for thirty seconds to a minute

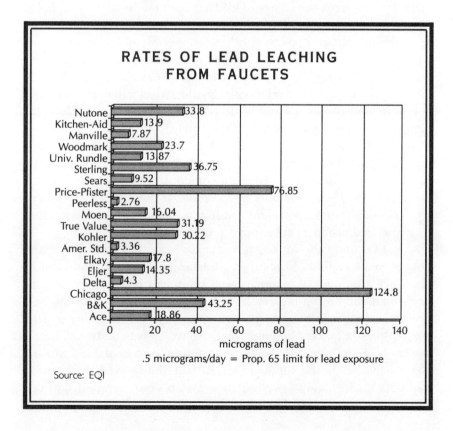

RATES OF LEAD LEACHING
FROM FAUCETS

Nutone 33.8
Kitchen-Aid 13.9
Manville 7.87
Woodmark 23.7
Univ. Rundle 13.87
Sterling 36.75
Sears 9.52
Price-Pfister 76.85
Peerless 2.76
Moen 16.04
True Value 31.19
Kohler 30.22
Amer. Std. 3.36
Elkay 17.8
Eljer 14.35
Delta 4.3
Chicago 124.8
B&K 43.25
Ace 18.86

micrograms of lead

.5 micrograms/day = Prop. 65 limit for lead exposure

Source: EQI

before drawing water for consumption. The common-sense advice is based on the fact that water sits in the system overnight, with more time to leach lead. When Dr. Maas tested the brass faucets for leaching, he let the water sit in the faucets for 16 hours, to mimic the overnight situation. But he also tested after letting the water sit for only two hours.

"In only three of 19 cases," Dr. Maas says, "was the 16-hour concentration significantly higher. These results clearly indicate that most lead is leached from brass faucets during the first two hours that water is stored in the faucets." What this means is that you should flush water from a faucet anytime it has been sitting for more than a few minutes, certainly if it's been an hour or more, as well as in the morning. (To conserve water, fill a bottle after flushing and keep it in the refrigerator for middle-of-the-night water calls. Water for morning coffee can be drawn the night before.)

The EQI study of faucet leaching actually offers a great deal of hope to homeowners. Most of the attention in terms of the role of the home water system as a source of lead has been on the solder that holds copper fittings together. The result is a sense of homeowner hopelessness. Tearing out and replacing all the copper plumbing in a house is a task and expense almost beyond comprehension. It's certainly not practical. But replacing the kitchen faucet is practical. It's relatively simple and inexpensive. And if replacing the faucet will cut the amount of lead in your drinking water by 30 percent, that alone could be sufficient to bring your water within safe standards.

If you are buying a new faucet, ask to see the manufacturer's catalog. This should list both the process used to make the faucet and the percent of lead it contains. The lead content of many faucets is much lower than the legal maximum of 8 percent. If the company refuses to give you this information, find a different manufacturer. Companies with low-lead products are happy to tell you about them.

The EQI study also looked at what may be the faucets of the future. They're made of plastic, and they've been around since the early 1980s. There are a number of manufacturers offering a broad range of both kitchen and bathroom faucets. Brian Camp, sales manager of Lifetime Faucets, based in Hot Springs, Arkansas, says his company started making plastic faucets because corrosive water was destroying brass faucets in many parts of the South. Lifetime gets its name from the lifetime guarantee the company gives. "We didn't even think about lead back then," Camp says, "but now we label our cartons 'lead-free,' and we're getting a lot of interest." Though plastic faucets do contain trace amounts of lead, left over from the manufacturing process, they leach far less lead than any brass faucet in EQI's California study.

It is possible to make metal faucets that don't leach lead. Of special note is the Lead Free dispensing faucet; EQI testing showed it leaches less lead than even the plastic models. It's made by a small start-up company, Lead Free Faucets, Inc., of Chagrin Falls, Ohio. President Walter Wright explains that he was working for a large company doing industrial copper alloy molding when he saw the application of a particular lead-free bronze alloy for use in faucets. Lead Free's first venture was a dispensing faucet for under-the-counter water filtration units, and it's now bringing on the market a device for dispensing hot and cold water. Entrepreneur Wright says he has a prototype kitchen faucet, but it may be a year or more—depending on how his business grows—before he can bring it to market. The Lead Free is one of two brass fixtures that will not require a Proposition 65 warning label; the other is the Swiss-made KWCdomo faucet.

EQI also tested three instant hot-water dispensers. These would seem like a parent's best friend, delivering formula-ready hot water on demand, perfect for that 2:00 A.M. bottle. Unfortunately, like any plumbing fixture that holds water, especially hot water, these units add lead to the water. In fairness, the ISE IN-SINKERATOR Hot-1 added only 0.4 ppb, but this is still lead *added* to that already in your water. Other units added significantly more. Your best bet is still to flush your tap and then heat *cold* water to make infant formula and cereal.

THE DANGER OF LEAD SOLDER

In June 1984, a blood-lead test run on a 24-month-old Massachusetts girl as part of a routine checkup turned up a blood-lead level of 42 μg/dl. A public health inspector went to the little girl's home and tested paint, inside and out. The home was new. The paint contained no lead. Furniture and toys were tested. Still no lead. The child was re-tested several times while the investigation went on. Lead levels dropped briefly, then rose to 45 μg/dl. Homes where the child visited or played were tested. Still no lead. Food and even yard soil were eliminated as sources. Finally, on one visit, the child's mother remarked that her daughter was allergic to milk and drank a lot of apple juice diluted with tap water. Tests on water drawn from the kitchen tap showed it carried 390 ppb of lead. Bathroom taps were almost as high. When the aerator-filter on the faucet was removed, flakes of loose solder fell out. Tests showed they were between 55 and 80 percent lead.

The child's mother was told to clean the faucet filters regularly* and to run her water for five minutes before using it for anything her daughter would consume. Within six months, the little girl's blood-lead level was down to 22 µg/dl. The case dramatized the danger of lead solder, and on January 1, 1986, Massachusetts instituted the nation's first ban on the use of lead solder in lines carrying drinking water.

Along with brass faucets, lead solder is a major contributor of lead to your home water supply. Look at the supply pipes (those are the little reddish brown ones leading to the shut-off valves) under your kitchen sink. If your house was built after 1950, or someone had the plumbing redone, the pipes are most likely copper. Sections of copper plumbing are connected with soldered fittings. The solder used was typically a tin-lead alloy, containing from 50 to 95 percent lead. Flux, a substance used to aid the flow of solder, also contains lead.

You've probably never looked at the inside of a soldered fitting, but the solder flows into the joint when it's heated (*sweated* is the technical term) and will often form a thin film over much of the interior surface. When your water's not flowing through your pipes, it's sitting on that film of lead. You can almost hear it leaching.

There's not much you can do about your existing plumbing, but you can police any new plumbing that's being installed. Shop carefully for any new or replacement faucets, especially for kitchen and bath (see preceding section), and make certain that copper pipe and fittings are joined with lead-free solder. Any reel of solder that you or your plumber uses should say "lead-free" or "safe for drinking water systems." If in doubt, ask the building inspector to test it, or scrape some solder off the pipes and test it yourself.

The EPA banned the use of lead solder in water supply systems in 1988, but lead solder is still available and too widely used. Check for yourself. Go into your local hardware store; I'll bet there's still lead solder sitting on the shelf even today. A lot of do-it-yourselfers end up using lead solder in their home improvement projects simply because that's what's on the shelf, and they don't know any better. If you're handy enough to be doing your own copper plumbing, be sure you're using lead-free solder.

---

*It's a good idea to remove the little strainers on the end of your kitchen and bathroom faucets from time to time and run the water for several minutes. Small pieces of solder occasionally collect on the strainers. Always do this after you have plumbing work done on your supply pipes; loose solder and other debris need to be flushed out.

Don't assume your plumber knows, or is obeying, the law regarding the use of leaded solder. Plumbers' resistance to change was driven home to me early in this book project. Two days after I delivered a chapter-by-chapter outline to my agent, I got an urgent phone call from her. I somehow knew she hadn't sold the book quite that quickly, and it turned out that she was in the middle of a remodeling project. While she was upstairs reading the outline of this chapter, the plumber was downstairs preparing to solder the pipes to her new kitchen. She asked if he was using lead-free solder. "Oh no, lady," he told her. "That stuff's no good. If I used no-lead solder, all these pipes would be leaking within a year."

The problem with hiring experienced people, my father was fond of saying, is that sometimes they're a bad experience. Certainly this plumber's experience was about 20 years out of date. Although early attempts to come up with a lead-free solder left a lot to be desired, the problem was solved years ago. John Moran, of Canfield Quality Solder, says the lead-free solders on the market today are far superior to the old leaded solders. His company markets a "100% Water Safe Solder" which has been tested to consistently withstand pressures of 10,000 psi (pounds per square inch). Lead-base solders tested out at 4,500 psi.

My agent's plumber was involved in risky business. Risky for her because she has small children, and because new solder releases lead at a far greater rate than fittings that have been in place for six years or more. Risky for the plumber, too, because the work was being done in New York City, which requires both plumbers and plumbing jobs to be licensed. Inspectors can test for lead by simply scraping some solder off with a knife, dropping it into a vial, and watching to see if the liquid changes color. Had an inspector shown up and tested the work in my agent's home, the test solution would have turned bright yellow. The job would have been condemned, and the plumber ordered to rip out and replace everything he'd installed. He would also have faced forfeiture of his license.

Given all that, if copper plumbing has been installed in your home anytime since 1986, you should probably test the solder for lead. (See appendix D for information on lead-test kits and services.) The EPA says that if the solder contains lead, you should "notify the plumber who did the work and request that he or she replace the lead solder with lead-free solder." You can try, but you should probably also be prepared to call your lawyer. One number you should definitely call is the state or local agency responsible for enforcing the Safe Drinking

Water Act in your locality. You can get that number from the people who supply your water.

CHECK YOUR HOME'S ELECTRICAL GROUNDS

Go to your electric box and trace the ground wire. If you don't know how to do this, ask the meter reader, or call in an electrician. If your home's electrical system is grounded to the water supply system, it can increase the rate of lead leaching. A licensed electrician will know whether the ground can be moved. *Do not attempt to move the ground yourself. An improperly grounded system can cause electric shock and can create a fire hazard.* Check your pipes for other wires that may be connected to them. Telephone lines are often grounded to plumbing systems. So are doorbells. Even this small amount of electric current traveling through the pipes will increase the rate of corrosion.

NATIONWIDE TESTING FOR LEAD IN WATER

The problem of lead in water is by no means limited to New York or the Northeast. In May 1993, the EPA released the results of lead tests taken in every large and medium public water system in the country. More than 800 systems, serving some 30 million people, reported lead concentrations above the federal action level of 15 ppb. Forty-two states, from Maine to Alaska and Florida to Hawaii, all reported elevated lead levels. Major cities included Boston, Chicago, Cleveland, Milwaukee, New York, Seattle, and Washington. Naturally corrosive groundwater in the Carolinas was responsible for their especially high lead levels; Charleston, South Carolina, at 165 ppb, had the highest levels among large water systems, and the midsize U.S. Marine Corps Camp LeJeune-Hadnot Point system in North Carolina reported a scary 484 ppb.

The EPA had tightened standards for lead in public drinking water in December 1992. It cut allowable lead levels from 50 to 15 ppb. At the same time, recognizing that there appears to be no safe threshold for lead, the EPA established a *goal* of zero ppb. Even this brought criticism from environmentalists, who testified before the House Energy and Commerce Subcommittee on Health and the Environment that the level should be set even lower, at 5 ppb. The argument for a lower allowable limit is bolstered by at least one study, which indicates that measurable neurological effects can be found with 10 ppb.

The test results reported by the EPA don't mean that every one of those 30 million people is drinking water with high levels of lead. The tests are designed to look for lead in likely places. The samples are taken in homes with lead plumbing or service lines, or with lead-soldered copper pipes. They are "first draw" tests, taken at the faucet after water has been sitting without flowing for at least six hours. If your city or town exceeded the federal action level but your home has old iron pipes or new plastic pipes—neither of which leach lead—or it's a new home with copper pipes joined with lead-free solder, you are probably not at risk.

EPA REQUIREMENTS FOR REDUCING EXPOSURE

If the water system in your city or town tested high, by now you should have gotten a notice from your water supplier, along with a brochure telling you steps you can take to reduce your exposure.* Public education is one of the first actions the EPA requires because simply flushing out the water that's been sitting in your pipes and faucets overnight (or while everyone's at work) can significantly cut the lead contamination in the water you drink. This is especially true if you live in a single-family home, where all the pipes in the house may hold only a couple of quarts of water. Even in a large apartment building, flushing will eliminate the lead contamination leached from your faucets.

Flushing the toilet or taking a shower in the morning will flush your supply pipes of water that's been sitting overnight. (Showering is okay; your body doesn't absorb lead through the skin.) You will still need to run each tap (kitchen and bath) for about thirty seconds to flush the water that sat in the faucet itself.

The ability of water to accumulate lead while sitting in pipes was demonstrated dramatically in Clewiston, Florida. The city initially reported lead levels of 166 ppb. It turned out that two-thirds of the city's water samples had been taken in vacant condominiums where the water had been sitting for months. When the city went back and retested,

*Don't assume that no news is good news. If you haven't received information from your water supplier, call and ask for results of testing under the EPA's "Lead and Copper Rule." More than 1,100 water systems nationwide had not completed their monitoring by the EPA deadline.

letting the water sit for only six hours, composite lead levels dropped 139 points. Remember that when you come back from your two-week vacation in Tahiti. Flush your pipes and faucets!

Although the sources of lead contamination lie mostly within private homes or apartment buildings—the water delivered by the public system is generally free of lead—it's just not practical or economically feasible for people to rip out and replace all of their supply pipes. When we discovered that our supply line was lead, I got estimates on replacing it. The cheapest was over $5,000. Then I realized that the old iron pipes inside the house had been replaced with copper at some point in time, and the soldered fittings were also adding lead to my water. I didn't even consider getting an estimate on that, and neither should you. You can buy a lot of bottles of water with the money it would cost to replace copper plumbing. (See discussion of bottled water later in this chapter.) Remember, your primary concern is reducing the exposure of your preschool child. Adults need to limit their exposure to lead by all *practical* means, but lead in drinking water is not, by itself, generally a threat to older children and adults.

Fortunately, there are cheaper, more sensible solutions than tearing out your plumbing. The ability of water to leach lead is governed in part by its pH and alkalinity. Low pH water is acidic, and we all know that acid is corrosive. Soft water is water that has a low mineral content. If the water doesn't have a lot of minerals, it has more room to pick up and carry lead. To reduce lead levels, the EPA requires water systems that test above 15 ppb to raise the pH and to add mineral compounds to the water. Compounds include lime or calcium carbonate, soda ash or sodium hydroxide (sodium hydroxide will raise the sodium level in the water, but not above the recommended limits for people on salt-restricted diets), calcium hydroxide, calcium oxide, and orthophosphate compounds. These chemicals are nontoxic and act to reduce the water's corrosiveness. They also deposit a mineral film on the inside of pipes which forms a barrier between the water and the lead that's in the plumbing components. These two factors, working in combination, can significantly cut the rate of leaching.

Hard water naturally coats pipes with a mineral film. That's why many old lead pipes and lead-soldered copper fittings that have been in place for six or eight years no longer pose a threat. The water runs through them without ever being exposed to the lead they contain.

The EPA requires that large water systems (serving more than 50,000 customers) have corrosion treatment systems in place by 1997, medium-sized systems by 1998, and the small systems that serve fewer than 3,300 must be treating their water by 1999 if their lead levels are above the magic 15 ppb. The cost of all of this is not terribly high and may actually save money in the long run. Reducing corrosion will reduce leaks and water main failures. Water will appear cleaner, too, because less rust and flaking metal will be carried to your tap. Too late to help us, New York City began adding calcium orthophosphate to its water in September 1992.

It's worth noting that while most drinking water supplies start out free of lead, a few systems do pick up lead at their source. The EPA requires those systems to remove the lead, usually through filtration or a reverse-osmosis system, so that water at the tap does not exceed 15 ppb.

If tinkering with the water's ability to leach lead doesn't get a system's levels below the magic 15 ppb, it becomes time for the backhoe and the bank loan. At this point, the EPA requires water systems to start replacing lead service lines. They have 15 years to complete the job, at a rate of 7 percent a year. Often, part of the service line is the property owner's responsibility. The water system is required to replace whatever part of the lead service line is theirs, and must offer to replace your part as well "at the building owner's expense." Check the cost, but this may turn out to be a good deal. When we were looking into the cost of replacing our service line, we discovered there were only two outfits in all of Brooklyn that handle this work. No surprise that they both quoted the same (astronomical) price to replace the line. If your service line is lead and it breaks or leaks, you probably won't be allowed to repair it. Most cities require that lead lines be replaced as they fail. Washington, D.C., has replaced almost 1,500 lead service lines in the past five years but estimates that more than 26,000 remain in service.

TESTING THE DRINKING WATER IN YOUR HOME

Ultimately, the only way to know if your drinking water contains lead is to test it. If your home gets water from a public system, ask if a free lead test is available. If it turns out you need to pay for the services of a water-testing lab, be advised that some use hard-sell scare tactics. The first one we called told us our water "was known to have bacteria" and a host of other nightmares in it, all of which the company would be only too happy to test for. Suddenly the cost went from $40 for a lead test to more than $250. Unless you have your own well, you don't need all that other stuff. Your water supplier already tests for everything except lead. We called a different lab. (See appendix C for information on finding a lab.)

You should actually test two samples of water. One should be a

WATER-TESTING LABS

The EQI lab in Asheville, North Carolina, has built an enormous drinking water data base by performing drinking water tests at cost. Their test kits are distributed by:

Clean Water Lead Testing
29½ Page Avenue
Asheville, NC 28801
($17.00/kit, includes S&H)

SAVE
P.O. Box 1723
FDR Station
New York, NY 10150
(718) 626-3936
($15.00/kit, plus $1.50/kit S&H)

Environmental Law Foundation
1736 Franklin Street, 7th Fl.
Oakland, CA 94612
(510) 208-4555
($15.00/kit, plus flat $1.50 S&H)

Each kit tests two samples (first and second draw). Turn-around time for results is approximately two weeks.

You can also refer to appendix C for a list of other labs that test water by mail, or contact your water supplier for a list of EPA-certified laboratories. The state agencies that recommend certified labs are listed in appendix D. You can also call the EPA Water Hotline, (800) 426-4791.

"first draw" sample. This should be done first thing in the morning, before anyone flushes a toilet and before any water is run from any tap. Draw water from the cold-water faucet in your kitchen, without letting any spill, and draw only the amount your particular lab calls for.

The second sample (second draw) should be taken after the faucet and the system has been flushed. Having the results of both tests will tell you your worst-case scenario (first draw) and whether flushing the system is sufficient to reduce lead levels to the point your water is safe to drink. If the "first draw" sample comes back below 15 ppb, you have nothing to worry about. If the first is above 15 but the second is below, make it a habit to let the water run before drawing water to drink or cook with, and consider replacing the faucet.

If the second sample comes back above 15 ppb, it means that flushing won't help. The simplest solution is to filter your drinking and cooking water or use bottled water from an approved source. "Approved source" means either your grocery store or a source (someone else's tap, a spring, whatever) that has been tested. Taking these measures is especially important for pregnant women and nursing mothers, with water used to make infant formula, and with water consumed by children under the age of seven.

SHOPPING FOR BOTTLED WATER

We used bottled water. I'm not a Perrier kind of guy, and it drives me nuts to pay a buck a gallon for something the city provides for less than a penny. New York City water tastes great too; I just can't find a practical (read cheap) way of getting city water past that lead snake in my basement and the faucet in the kitchen. It especially galled me when I discovered that a lot of bottled water starts out as city tap water!

Shopping for water, I've come to conclude, is worse than shopping for a car. At least with a car, you can choose between the red one or the blue one. Go to the water section, and there's row upon row of identical bottles all filled with clear liquid. I'm talking primarily about "bulk or still" water, sold in one- to five-gallon bottles, as opposed to the panoply of flavored and unflavored soda waters, sparkling waters, seltzers, and mineral waters that are classified as "specialty waters."

The important thing to know is that *all* bottled water should be as lead-free as water can be. While public drinking water is regulated by the EPA, drinking water bottled for inter-state sale comes under FDA

ACTING ON TEST RESULTS

FIRST DRAW	SECOND DRAW	ACTION*
Less than 15 ppb	Less than 15 ppb	You do not have a lead problem. No action is necessary.
More than 15 ppb	Less than 15 ppb	Flush the faucet each time you use it; replace the faucet.
More than 15 ppb	More than 15 ppb	Use bottled water; filter or purify your water; confer with your water supplier; replace lead sources in your home plumbing system.

*These actions are for drinking water to be consumed by pregnant or nursing mothers, infants, toddlers, and children up to age seven. Adults are not at risk until lead levels in water exceed 180 ppb.

regulation. (Bottled water sold locally comes under state regulation.) After being criticized by the General Accounting Office (GAO) for lax regulation, the FDA recently set stringent new standards for lead in bottled water. It lowered the allowable levels to 5 ppb (one-third of what the EPA has set for public drinking water). The International Bottled Water Association (IBWA), which represents about 85 percent of the bottled water sold in the United States, supported the change wholeheartedly. "In reality," says IBWA Vice President Lisa Prats, "bottled water could meet any measurable limits you could set for lead. It's just not there."

Water, as I've said before, does not naturally contain lead. Water bottling companies are prohibited from letting their water touch anything made with lead. Pipes and tanks in a bottling plant are made of either stainless steel or PVC plastic. There is no lead to get into the water. The companies that bottle city water—the tip-off on the label is "purified drinking water"—go through an elaborate filtration, purification, and disinfection process before they add back some minerals and put it in a plastic jug with a nature scene on the label. (They add back the minerals because not many people enjoy truly pure H_2O; it's tasteless.) "Purified drinking water" is as close to absolutely lead-free as you can get.

The problem with bottled water is that although the FDA has set excellent standards, it does little to monitor them. The GAO report found that plants were rarely inspected, and bottlers were not required to report test results to the FDA. IBWA members are required to regularly conduct testing that goes far beyond FDA requirements. In addition, association members agree to let an independent testing group conduct unannounced plant inspections. You can find out if your preferred brand of water is bottled by an IBWA member by calling (800)-WATER-11, that is, (800) 928-3711.

Strolling the water aisle and reading labels, I was struck that no one had emblazoned "lead-free" across the label. This, after all, is not an industry that is shy in its advertising. There was "Baby's First Spring Water," from Beech-Nut at an outrageous $1.09 a quart, but it said not a word about lead. In fact, of the 15 brands for sale, only two even mentioned lead, and one of them was the $0.59-per-gallon Key Food store brand. In tiny print, it said its lead content was "less than 0.0001 mg/l." This translates into less than one-tenth of a part per billion, but that's still not good enough to be called "lead-free." Technology cannot measure zero. And when it comes to things people eat and drink, zero doesn't mean less than some gazillionth part per billion; zero means zero. Nevertheless, I still don't understand why more bottled waters don't include some statement about lead.

WATER FILTERS AND PURIFIERS

Filtering or purifying your water at home is a big deal. The equipment can be expensive. It can be expensive to run and maintain. The equipment can take up a lot of space. You have to filter at each tap. You have to remember to change whatever is filtering the water. And not all filters will filter out lead.

More than 400 companies have jumped into this field, and many of them survive by hyping fear. The Better Business Bureau says complaints have skyrocketed. *Consumer Reports* magazine, which published a thorough report on this industry in its January 1990 issue, summed up the situation as follows: "Many people buy equipment they don't need to cure a problem that never existed." It's worth a trip to the library to look at this report before you confront a water treatment salesman.

If you decide you must have filtration or purification equipment, prepare yourself. Make sure you have a certified test of your water and get ready for the hard sell. By all means, don't rely on the salesman to test your water for you; it will be the most expensive "free" test you've ever gotten. Some salesmen charge exorbitant fees for testing, and when you gasp, they suggest that "for a few dollars more," you can have their whiz-bang filter installed. Our local Culligan dealer runs newspaper ads touting lead tests for water. Their test costs $100 plus shipping and handling. If your only concern is lead, make sure the equipment you're getting will in fact remove lead, and don't get talked or panicked into buying more than you need.

Forget about those toy filters that mount on the end of the faucet— they are useless. You still have a number of systems to choose between. Under-the-sink systems are the most elegant. They are also the bulkiest and most expensive, involving the expense of both equipment and installation. They are plumbed directly into your cold-water supply, and, to avoid lead contamination from your sink faucet, they must have their own tap.

Countertop systems that attach to your existing faucet are less expensive but are, to my eye, clumsy. Not only do they take up counter space, they also have the added annoyance of hoses to get in the way. These are midpriced units to buy, and cost nothing to install.

In addition to selecting a filter system, you have to choose a type of filter. Sand or sediment filters *do not* remove lead from water. However, you may need to install one before whatever else you use, so sediments don't clog it. Only a few carbon filters remove lead; most do not. Activated alumina is perhaps the best filter for removing lead. *Consumer Reports* tested and reported favorably on the "Selecto Lead Out" alumina filter. It is also listed by NSF.

NSF, formerly the National Sanitation Foundation, is a private, independent, not-for-profit, and well-respected organization that works with government and industry to solve public health and environmental safety problems. Manufacturers voluntarily submit equipment to NSF for testing. If the equipment—in this case, filters and reverse-osmosis (R-O) units—does what it says it will do, and does it to established standards, the equipment gets an NSF listing. You get peace of mind.

Be sure the specific unit you're considering is NSF rated. When I called Culligan, I got a packet of information, including NSF material.

It took a close reading to realize that Culligan's System 201 lead filter ($360, installed) is not NSF listed. The company can include NSF material because its H-83 reverse-osmosis unit ($985, installed) is NSF listed. You can obtain a list of approved filters from NSF International, 3475 Plymouth Road, P. O. Box 130140, Ann Arbor, Michigan 48113-0140, (313) 769-8010, fax: (313) 769-0109.

After you've purchased a filter, be sure to clean or replace it on schedule. If you don't, it not only stops filtering but can become a breeding ground for bacteria.

Water distillers sit on the counter, boil the water, leaving lead and other contaminants in the boiling chamber, and then condense the steam, turning it into pure if tasteless water. Your iron will love it. Your electric bill won't. Distillers are noisy, obviously hot, and very slow.

The hi-tech approach to clean water is a reverse-osmosis system. R-O systems are used aboard ships, along the Florida coast, and in the Persian Gulf to desalinate seawater. To put it simply: R-O systems purify water, removing everything including minerals and heavy metals. They do an excellent job of removing lead. The better ones, like the under-sink filter system, are expensive, take a lot of room, require installation (including a sediment filter), and must have their own tap. There are also smaller countertop units. R-O units are terribly wasteful of water. Only 10 to 25 percent of the water entering the unit is purified; the rest goes down the drain. *Consumer Reports* tested 16 units. On average, they wasted 13 gallons of water a day. One, however, sent 40 gallons a day down the drain—some 14,000 gallons a year. One final knock: By removing all minerals from the water, R-O units leave it pretty tasteless.

If I sound down on the fancy expensive systems, I am. They do not seem a practical or economical answer for most people with the problem of lead in their drinking water. In the first place, public drinking water suppliers are working to bring lead levels down. The problem may go away without your doing anything. Buy bottled water or a countertop unit to use until levels come down or your child turns seven. Most high readings can be avoided by flushing the system. If that's too much bother, replace the kitchen faucet with one that leaches at very low levels. That's a onetime fix, with no perpetual maintenance costs or headaches. Only if flushing the system or replacing the faucets doesn't do the job should you consider installing filtration. Even then, you may be better off with a countertop unit or just buying bottled water. The annual cost of having filters replaced runs from $75 to $250; you can buy a lot of store-brand water for that money.

A SIMPLE COUNTERTOP FILTER

The simplest water filters are the ones that work like a drip coffee-maker. You pour water into the top. It runs through the filter into a carafe that can be stored in the refrigerator. The only countertop unit listed by the NSF for lead reduction is the Canadian Brita Water Filtering Pitcher. I tried one out. It's simple and effective. It takes about 15 minutes to make two quarts of water. You replenish as you use. The entire filter/pitcher unit goes in the frig.

The Brita uses a charcoal/ion exchange/silver filter cartridge. During NSF testing, the filter removed from 91 to 98 percent of the lead in the test water. Tests on water laced with 150 ppb lead produced an end product containing only 3 to 6 ppb, well below the EPA action level of 15 ppb. The unit is also listed for the removal of other metals, odor, chlorine, sediment, and bacteriological effects. The Brita should never be used to filter hot water, and the company says it "is only to be used with municipally treated tap water or well water that is regularly tested to be microbiologically safe." In other words, expect a lot, but not miracles.

Replacement filter cartridges cost $8 by mail, less in some discount stores. Brita says the filter is good for 35 gallons of water. That works out to about 23¢ a gallon, well below the cost of buying bottled water. The pitcher takes slightly less space in the frig than a gallon bottle, plus you don't have to schlep the water from the store.

PRIVATE WATER SUPPLIES

So far, we have talked about drinking water standards of 15 ppb, and lead contamination ranging up to several hundred parts per billion. One family found itself drinking water containing *20,000 ppb*.

It happened in rural New England. The family moved into a new mobile home and drilled a shallow well to supply their drinking water. Not long after, their three-year-old child was tested for lead poisoning as part of a required screening program. The test showed blood-lead levels over 50 µg/dl, and the child was hospitalized for chelation treatment (see chapter 2). Because the trailer was brand-new, health inspectors turned quickly to the water. It was then they found the extraordinary contamination.

The lead contamination was eventually traced to a previous owner of the property, who had been smelting lead out of scrap telephone boxes. The man carried out the smelting operation in open pits dug in the ground. Molten lead permeated the ground and contaminated the groundwater below. The well was immediately sealed. The family eventually had to move, and the property is now an official hazardous waste site.

People who have their own wells or who share a water supply with neighbors are at special risk. They aren't covered by the Safe Drinking Water Act, and by and large, they have sole responsibility for the quality of the water their families drink. If this is how you get your water, by all means test it (and not just for lead).

Most lead in drinking water gets there after the water enters your house. So start by testing your water at the tap. Test both "first draw" and after flushing the faucet. If the reading is still over 15 ppb after flushing pipes and taps, retest the water at the well-head or other source. If the water at the source is over 15 ppb, you have a serious problem and may need to bring in outside experts, starting perhaps with the local health department.

Four major manufacturers of submersible deep-well water pumps were recently sued by the California attorney general and the Natural Resources Defense Council because their pumps leached excessive levels of lead. The lead was leaching from brass and bronze parts within pumps made by Goulds Pump, Aermotor, Sta-Rite and F. E. Myer. At the same time, the EPA recommended that all private well owners test their water for lead, and suggested that families with newly installed pumps—less than one year old—use bottled water for children until their drinking water could be tested.

Older pumps are not considered to be a hazard, since the rate of lead leaching falls off sharply over time. The National Ground Water Association says almost half a million submersible pumps were sold in the United States in 1993. Nearly 12 million households, two-thirds of them in the South and Midwest, drink private well water. Not all deep-well pumps leach lead. California tested pumps manufactured by Grundfos and found them to be lead-free.

If your water source is free of lead contamination, you need to consider installing a calcite filter or some other corrosion control system. Calcite filters should be installed in the system before the water gets to the source(s) of lead contamination. Remember that calcite filters require maintenance.

If you have a water softener to remove iron, make sure it's not connected to the cold-water side of your supply system. Soft water is corrosive, and a water softener can increase the ability of water to leach lead. You only need to soften the hot water to be able to make soap suds.

If you have a lead rainwater collection system, common in Hawaii and the Florida Keys, or a lead-lined cistern as is often found outside old farmhouses, the lead levels of your water may be very high, and that part of the water system should be replaced.

7

FOOD AND DRINK

There is no margin of safety for kids.

—*Dr. John Rosen*
Montefiore Medical Center

CYNTHIA MEJIA, a dark-haired little girl with big eyes and a beautiful smile, found herself at the center of a health detective story that led to a national food recall.

It began with a routine twelve-month blood-lead test. Cynthia's blood-lead level was 36 μg/dl, three and a half times the threshold level. The results were reported to the San Diego County Health Department. When the little girl's parents were contacted, they said they'd just moved from a house that had badly peeling paint, but their new home was in good condition. The Health Department suggested a follow-up blood test to see if the family's move had brought Cynthia's lead level down. The second test, one month after the first, saw her lead level drop two points; not much, but at least it was going down. Another test was scheduled for three months later. Cynthia was nearly a year and a half old and had captivated everyone around her. The test results came back. Her blood-lead level was again 36 μg/dl. It could not be the paint at her old home.

Public health nurse Martha Bartzen was sent to visit the Mejias. Her job was to be a detective, to conduct an environmental survey, looking for clues that would point her to the source of the lead that was poisoning Cynthia. The little girl's mother and father showed Nurse Bartzen around the house and around the neighborhood. The home was neat and well maintained. There was no lead paint inside, no peeling paint outside. The soil outside did not contain lead, and the water at the tap was okay. There were no ceramic pots in the house and no lead-based industry in the area. No one else in the neighborhood had reported lead poisoning.

Cynthia was the Mejias' first child, and her mother, Elva, was anxious to do everything right for her daughter. "Look," she told the nurse, opening a kitchen pantry, "I even give her fruit juice all the time to make her healthy." The pantry was stocked with assorted cans of fruit juices and nectars. The juices all carried the Jumex label, a popular brand imported from Mexico and sold throughout the Southwest. Cynthia drank three cans a day. On a hunch, Nurse Bartzen asked to take one of the cans.

She sent the can of juice to an FDA laboratory. When the lab tested the juice, it was found to be loaded with lead. The cans were soldered with lead solder, and the lead was leached out by the acid in the fruit juices. In July 1992, the FDA announced a national recall of Jumex brand fruit nectar and pineapple juices. (The recall was for 12-ounce cans whose numerical code ended in 2084 or lower. Other Jumex products were packaged in cans with welded side seams and were not involved.)

Cynthia became the star of the local evening news. Her parents agreed to take their story public so others could be warned about the dangers of lead. Cynthia was fortunate. Mandatory blood testing revealed her lead poisoning. The toxic fruit juice was removed from her diet, and the lead level in her blood quickly declined, down eight points after one month, another nine points after three months, and ultimately back to an acceptable level of 7 µg/dl. Her motor, language, and social skills have all been monitored and checked off "OK."

Lead poisoning has been traced to food and drink for centuries. Lead cooking and storage vessels were the cause of mass poisonings in Europe. At the turn of the century, in Philadelphia, large numbers of people were poisoned by bakers using lead chromate as a food coloring in baked goods. Until recently, America's food supply contained significant levels of lead. The FDA tracks what it calls "market basket" data, information used to estimate the total lead intake through food. In 1982, the average two-year-old child ingested from a combination of sources some 30 µg/dl of lead every day. That figure is down significantly, owing to the removal of lead from gasoline and discontinuing the use of lead soldered cans. Lead poisoning involving large numbers of people is also mercifully a thing of the past, but health officials are still seeing whole families acutely poisoned by lead they've consumed at the table, and there is still much that can be done to eliminate lead from our daily bread.

Simply by eating, drinking, and breathing, we still accumulate a blood-lead level of roughly 6 μg/dl. We cannot, as individuals, completely control this. Lead is a pervasive pollutant of the environment. However, there are things we can do to reduce that exposure. Our concern here is with the storage, preparation, and serving of what we eat and drink. We'll also talk about foods you may grow yourself, and a special risk faced by people, especially children and pregnant and nursing women, who are allergic to milk.

CHINA AND POTTERY

How many coffee mugs do you have in the house and at work? Glazed ceramics, from coffee mugs to fine china, are ubiquitous in our life. Almost everyone uses some kind of glazed pottery product, and most of us use them frequently. Because many contain lead, glazed ceramics are one of the last significant sources of lead in the American diet.

The first place to look for lead is in the glaze. Glaze has been used to coat, color, and decorate pottery and china for centuries. Made from powdered glass and various oxides, glaze is applied to the surface of an object and then fired—heated until it melts and bonds to form a hard, smooth, nonporous surface that is easily cleaned. Lead oxide was commonly used because it lowers the melting point of the glaze and makes it flow better. But improperly fired, lead-oxide glaze can be deadly, leaching its lead into food and drink.

There's a second possible source of lead in ceramics. Lead pigments are often used to provide color in the design. Lead-pigment colors hold their brilliance, so bright colors in a china pattern are often a tip-off to the presence of lead. However, the mere presence of lead does not mean there's a hazard. Lead-pigment designs can be and often are protected in such a way that the lead cannot leach out. The trick is knowing which dishes are safe.

The FDA first placed limits on the use of lead in ceramic-ware products, including pottery and china dishes, in 1970. The limits were lowered in 1980 and again in 1991, but as we learn more about the risks of low-level lead exposure, what was considered a safe level yesterday is unacceptable today, and the FDA may again reconsider and toughen the federal regulations. In the meantime, stringent California standards are coming to govern most products produced for national distribution.

Despite more than 20 years of regulation, isolated cases of severe lead poisoning from ceramics still occur. In 1987, seven people in a family from Westchester County, New York, were poisoned by a homemade fermented beverage stored in a Mexican ceramic bean jug. Their blood-lead levels ranged from 35 to 70 μg/dl, and three people had to be hospitalized for chelation therapy. The jug was tested; it had a lead content of 730 ppm. In 1973, several people living at an Oregon commune were severely poisoned by drinking plum wine made in a glazed vat. Their blood-lead levels reached as high as 98 μg/dl. In another case of multiple exposure, five members of a California family were poisoned by orange juice stored in a Mexican earthenware jug.

U.S. Customs intercepts suspect shipments of pottery and china and automatically holds them until the importer or distributor can prove they meet FDA standards. However, government resources are severely limited, and the safety net is thin indeed. Shipments are checked on the basis of origin, often on a village-by-village basis. Out of an estimated one and a half billion pieces of china sold annually in the United States, in 1989 (the last year for which it would reveal numbers), the federal government laboratory-tested just 900 pieces. A lot slips through. In a 1985 study, 67 pieces of Mexican glazed pottery obtained in the United States were tested for lead leaching. More than half exceeded even the relatively high FDA limits of the time. More than a quarter of the items released over 100 ppm lead. The worst tested at 9,900 ppm.

Mexico is by no means the only source of lead-bearing products entering the country (see list). The Environmental Defense Fund (EDF) tested a hand-painted French china plate purchased at New York's Tiffany and Company. The china was made to order for Tiffany's Private Stock line, whose average price for a five-piece setting of dinnerware was more than $1,000. When the EDF tested the plate, it leached lead at more than 200 times the FDA limit. It was the highest lead-leaching result the EDF had seen in a year of testing. When made aware of the lead levels, Tiffany sent letters to every registered owner of the Private Stock dinnerware warning of the danger and providing a merchandise credit if the products were returned. Clearly, though, neither price nor reputable source is an absolute guarantee of safety from lead poisoning. Only pattern-by-pattern testing can accomplish that.

Part of the problem is that because its testing program is limited by

PLACES KNOWN TO EXPORT CERAMICS WITH LEAD

The Maryland Department of the Environment reports that china and ceramic items from the following places may contain leaded glazes or decoration:

China	France	Hong Kong	India
Italy	Netherlands	Macao	Mexico
Morocco	Spain	North Korea	Portugal
Puerto Rico			

This list shouldn't be considered all-inclusive; don't assume that items from a place not on this list are free of lead glaze.

lack of funds, the government relies on a lot of assumptions. It assumes that white china is free of dangerous lead levels, and it concentrates on highly decorated ceramics imported from areas known to produce lead-leaching products. The FDA tests almost no domestic china. Yet the EDF, which has tested thousands of patterns, domestic and import, high end and low, decorated and white, has found there are no safe assumptions. Some white china has dangerous lead glaze; some brightly colored imports leach almost no lead, and there are patterns from well-known American manufacturers that leach considerable amounts.

There is one thing you can safely assume: When manufacturers or importers mark an object "For decorative use only," they mean it. They're telling you flat-out the plate or bowl or cup is *not safe to use with food or drink*. The warning is a red flag; dishes and other ceramic objects made and sold as art objects or as souvenirs are exempt from FDA standards for lead. That warning, by the way, must be a permanent part of the item—it cannot be a sticker—for it to qualify as a souvenir or art object; moreover, the ceramic cannot be part of a set. If it is an eight-inch dish, there cannot be a ten-inch dish, or a cup, and so forth. *Don't buy souvenir ceramic cups for your child to drink from.*

Even if a decorative plate or porcelain doesn't contain the danger warning, *avoid using it for food.* The highest lead level ever tested in

California, higher even than the bean pot mentioned earlier, was a piece of enameled porcelain. Officials explain that it was imported as plain white porcelain, stamped simply "Made in China," and then was enameled here. It was sold without any warning as to its lead content.

In addition to the problems regulating imports, it's virtually impossible to regulate the flow of souvenirs and personal belongings brought into the country by tourists and immigrants. You should be especially wary of any imported product not purchased from a reputable retailer. Tag-sale and street-vendor purchases as well as gifts and souvenirs from abroad are fine as decoration; just don't use them to serve or store food.

There's another source of high-risk ceramics here at home. These are the beautiful dishes and bowls and pitchers made by craftspeople and sold everywhere from craft fairs to specialty shops. They also include similar objects made by hobbyists for home use or gift giving. Uneven quality control or improper firing can result in a product that will leach high levels of lead. Don't use a glazed crafts product for storing or serving food unless it is certified lead-free. More and more craftspeople are turning to lead-free glazes and clearly advertise they've done so. Be especially careful with glazed mugs, cups, and teapots: Hot liquids leach lead at a much higher rate. *One of the worst things you can do is microwave coffee in a lead-glazed mug.*

The final area of concern for high-risk lead leaching is heirlooms, the dishes and other objects that have been passed down in the family—or bought in an antique store. Pre-1970 glazes should be assumed to have higher levels of leachable lead. Most of these dishes can be used, but you need to take certain precautions, which we'll get into below. However, dishes with glaze that is very worn or that has chipped or cracked are an even higher risk and shouldn't be used.

WHICH DISHES ARE THE BEST TO USE?

The risk of high-dose lead poisoning from dishes and food containers is mercifully low—thanks to regulation, education, and the threat to manufacturers of being sued. More common is the risk of low-level poisoning, the cumulative effect of consuming food that leaches minute amounts of lead from everyday dishes. That risk can vary significantly. The EDF, which tested hundreds of china samples, reports that the results varied, from best to worst, by a factor of 20,000. What to do?

First, there are some dishes you don't have to worry about. The unbreakable plastic dishes designed for use by children can be assumed to be safe. They contain no glaze, and the color and design are an integral part of the dish or cup. Glass dishes do not have glaze on them. Clear plates, cups, mugs, pitchers, bowls, and so on, are almost certainly lead-free unless they have been painted or carry decals. (This statement does not apply to crystal. See discussion later in the chapter.) Stoneware dishes are not lead glazed. Like glass, if they don't have decals or painted designs, you may assume they are lead-free.

If you're purchasing china and other ceramics new, choose a lead-free or low-lead product. This is especially true if you're selecting wedding china or some other object you expect to use through child-bearing and child-raising years. Products that are totally lead-free are starting to show up in the marketplace. One of the pioneers in changing to lead-free glaze has been the Hall China Company, which manufactures restaurant and institutional china; everything it makes now boasts lead-free glaze. (Incidentally, the china used in the White House dining room, made by Pickard, is totally lead-free.)

The selection of low-lead products is wider. Many companies have been producing low-lead ceramicware for years. Corningware, Corelle, and Pyrex (all made by Corning Consumer Products) have been low- or no-lead for years. More and more manufacturers are modifying their lines to meet the new California Proposition 65 standards. They grew out of a California suit against twelve major china manufacturers. The Prop. 65 standards set lead-leaching limits far below the national FDA limits. While it is still legal to sell a china pattern in California as long as it meets FDA standards, patterns that exceed the Prop. 65 limits must bear a triangular yellow sticker and carry the following health warning: "This product will expose you to lead, a chemical known to the State of California to cause birth defects or other reproductive harm."

David Roe, senior attorney for the Environmental Defense Fund, who helped bring the Prop. 65 suit, says one result has been a very strong move on the part of industry to remove lead from product lines. Settlement of the suit committed manufacturers to a 50 percent reduction in overall lead levels. Some have developed new processes to ensure that lead pigments in their design are sandwiched beneath a protective coating; others are moving completely away from lead pigments. Corning, even though its consumer products did not require the Prop. 65 warning, has worked with its suppliers to completely eliminate both lead and cadmium from enamels and glazes on surfaces that come into contact with food or drink. Other companies have either redesigned or withdrawn problem patterns.

The federal government may be on the verge of getting an important new tool for policing low-level lead violations. Lab-testing china in any volume is both time-consuming and expensive. Yet there has been no reliable field test for screening low-level leaching. That seems about to change. Michael Kashtock, chief of the FDA's Regulations and Enforcement Branch, is currently measuring the effectiveness of a newly developed field test. "This will let us do quick, rapid screening at the dock," he said. "If this works, it will let us detect samples that are problems at the low end of the scale."

Kashtock explains that some manufacturers have quality-control problems. Most of their china meets federal standards, but 10 or 20 percent of what they produce exceeds the lead limit. The ability to catch this problem in the field will put tremendous pressure on the china makers to tighten up. If an offending piece of china is caught, the manufacturer goes on detention status. The company is then subjected to the ultimate federal penalty—paperwork and red tape.

When shopping for china, ask the department or store manager if the pattern you're considering has been tested for lead leaching, and what the lead level is, for both plates and bowls. (Ask for the manufacturer's phone number and contact the company directly if you are not satisfied with the store manager's reliability.) Don't be fooled by such statements as: This china is perfectly legal; it meets federal standards; it's been inspected by the FDA; it meets the California Tableware standards, or it meets the California Prop. 65 standards. A salesman can honestly make any one of these statements about china that will leach lead. Ask whether the dish would require a warning if sold in California. If it does, and it's not one of those patterns with Christmas trees and holly berries that you'll use only once a year, don't buy it. The EDF and the California attorney general have compiled a list of china patterns that do not require warning labels under California's Prop. 65 lead exposure standards. It is available free from the EDF (see appendix B for address).

But what if you already own china? You can make some assumptions. White china is acknowledged to have fewer lead problems than colorful, highly decorated china (although many brightly decorated patterns do meet the California standards). Rim patterns are safer than patterns whose decoration and color extends onto the food-surface area of the plate or bowl. Be especially leery of using handcrafted mugs with a colored pattern on the inside. And watch out for any pattern whose decoration is on top of the glaze—you run the risk of lead leaching from the pigment as well as from the glaze.

LEAD-LEACHING STANDARDS FOR CHINA

ITEM	U.S. FDA STANDARDS	CALIF. STANDARDS
Plates	3.0 ppm	0.226 ppm
Small hollowware*	2.0 ppm	0.10 ppm
Large hollowware*	1.0 ppm	0.10 ppm
Cups/mugs†	0.5 ppm	0.10 ppm
Pitchers†	0.5 ppm	0.10 ppm

*Defined as anything with a depth greater than half an inch.

†Standards revised as of November 1991. *

If you know who manufactured your china, contact the company and ask questions, just as if you were buying new. You may get lucky, especially if your pattern is not too old; your manufacturer may be able to tell you the test results on your pattern. Ask for specific numbers; you are looking for the lead-leaching rate. Compare the figures you're given with both the FDA cut-off numbers and the California standards (see table). Be prepared for the same evasive dance that customers of new china get.

Our wedding china is Buchanan by Lenox. When I called Lenox customer service, I reached a voice oozing helpfulness and confidence. I was told with assurance, "Lenox has been testing their china for years and it's all well within both federal Food and Drug Administration guidelines and the California Tableware Safety standards."

"Does it meet the California Prop. 65 standards?" I asked.

"Oh, you must be from California," purred the voice. "California requires stickers on *all* pieces of china no matter what. It doesn't mean it's dangerous or you can't eat off it; it's just there to let you know there's lead in the plate."

I bit my tongue and pressed on, "Do you by chance have the test results on Buchanan?"

After a pause to look them up, she said, "I found your test results. Now, the FDA standards are 3.0 ppm, and the average of all pieces of Buchanan was 0.8 ppm."

Give Lenox an "A" for obfuscation. Compared to the FDA's 3.0, the 0.8 average sounds pretty benign. Unfortunately, averages don't count. The 3.0 FDA standard is only for plates. How about the teacups? The FDA cutoff there is 0.5; on average, then, my cups are over the limit. As for saying that California requires a sticker on all china, that's simply not true. There are many patterns of lead-free and low-lead china that don't need warning stickers in California. Lenox needs a warning sticker on its Buchanan pattern in California because it leaches anywhere from four to eight times the amount of lead allowed under Prop. 65 standards. When you talk to the china companies, arm yourself with enough facts to be able to judge the meaning of their answers.

TESTING YOUR CHINA

You can test your china yourself, but understand that tests you do at home will only alert you to high-risk china. They cannot measure the low-level leaching which can be cumulatively dangerous, depending on use. They can also give you a false negative, failing completely to detect low levels of lead. If a home lead test on china comes up positive, it means you shouldn't use the china; if it comes up negative, it doesn't tell you much of anything. (A list of suppliers of do-it-yourself lead-test kits is included in appendix H.)

Be sure to test several pieces of your china. It may not have all been purchased at the same time, and even china purchased as a set may have to be made up of several different manufacturing lots. Different lots can leach lead at different rates, depending on how they were fired.

Commercial laboratories that test for lead in paint will often test china for you. Your state agency lead office (see appendix D) should be able to recommend a laboratory in your area. However, commercial testing is expensive, running from $25 to $125 per item, and one type of analysis requires that the dish be chipped or broken to be tested!

HOW TO USE YOUR CHINA SAFELY

In the end, the safe use of your china may come down to risk elimination. Or at least minimization. How you use your china and how often you use it can significantly affect the level of lead it imparts to your food.

If you have china that you know or suspect leaches lead at a low rate (in the California-warning-level range), don't use it to serve food to infants and toddlers, and don't use it yourself everyday. *Don't ever*

Lead leaching is affected by several factors:

- Frequency of use
- Acidity of drink or food
- Temperature of drink or food
- Length of time in contact

store food or liquid (especially acidic juices) in anything ceramic; the longer the food is in contact with the surface, the more lead it will leach out. Acidic foods will leach lead faster than bland foods. Here's a partial list of acidic food and drink:

alcohol	salad dressings
apple juice	salsa
apple sauce	sauerkraut
citrus juices	soy sauce
coffee	spaghetti sauce
cola drinks	tea
fermented beverages	tomatoes
grapefruit juice	vinegar
ketchup	wine
orange juice	

Heat will also increase the rate of leaching, so *don't heat food in ceramic or china dishes.*

Any food left in contact with a lead-leaching ceramic long enough will pick up lead. So use suspect dishes wisely and sparingly. If you can't bring yourself to return your hand-painted Private Stock bowl to Tiffany's, use it only occasionally, and serve dry chips or crackers in it instead of hot toddy.

Remember that lead accumulates in the body, especially in children, so you want to look first at the ceramics you use most frequently. Low-level lead leaching from the bowl in which you serve hot cereal to your toddler all winter is a far greater threat than higher-level leaching from the heirloom china you use only on holidays. The mug you drink coffee from several times a day, every day of the week, is of more concern than the soup dishes you may use once a month (especially if the mug goes in the microwave for reheating). Everyday dishes, cups, and mugs should be lead-free or low lead. Suspect dishes should be reserved for occasional use. Decorative dishes shouldn't ever be used for food.

As for our Lenox china, we still use it, though sparingly. It recently graced our Thanksgiving dinner table, but Matthew and his cousin Alex ate their turkey and fixings from plastic Thomas-the-Tank-Engine plates. That seemed the commonsense thing to do.

CRYSTAL

Lead is what makes the difference between ordinary glass and fine crystal. Lead, or more technically lead oxide, was first introduced into glass late in the seventeenth century, when English glass makers produced what they called flint glass. The lead oxide imparted extraordinary brilliance and clarity. At the same time, it softened the glass, making it easier to cut patterns into everything from chalices to decanters. When the Crown imposed an excise tax, the glass companies established factories in a number of Irish cities including Waterford. Which brings us to all those bridal magazine advertisements and the agony/ecstacy of the Bridal Registry, when in a rush of romance you mix and match until you've chosen the patterns of china and silver and crystal that will likely define festive dining for the rest of your life.

Since lead content equates to quality, you can usually find out just how much lead the crystal contains by looking closely at the magazine ads or at those little stickers on the bottoms of display merchandise. Lead-oxide content in crystal can range as high as 35 percent, though most is 24 percent. (The percentage in optical instrument glass often is double the latter figure, producing a glass of incredible clarity, but which is soft and easily scratched.)

If your new crystal comes with a warning not to put it in the dishwasher, don't think the manufacturer is worried about the stemware being broken. The warning is given because the high temperatures and prolonged washing cycles in dishwashers can increase the hazard of lead leaching. Some dishwashers have a "china-crystal" cycle. This cycle is gentler, so as not to break delicate items. But there is no change in the water temperature, and it's still best to hand-wash your crystal stemware.

Alcohol will gradually leach lead from crystal. So will the acids in tomato and fruit juices. This doesn't mean you have to lock the crystal away and serve the boss wine in a paper cup. The leaching process is slow, especially when the liquid is cool. Since most of us don't drink from crystal at every meal, the occasional use of crystal stemware poses little threat.

The danger comes when liquids are stored in crystal containers, especially antiques, for a prolonged period. My mother always kept a beautiful cut-crystal decanter of cream sherry in our dining room. It was more for decoration than libation, so the sherry sat there at room temperature for months on end, quietly acquiring an unwanted additive of lead.

The state of California recently sued a number of crystal decanter manufacturers under Prop. 65. Tests showed that anywhere from 200 to 800 ppb of lead would leach out in a 24-hour period. That may not sound like much, but two ounces of brandy stored for a day in an 800 ppb decanter will give you *100 times* the maximum amount of lead you're supposed to get in a day. Consider that the brandy may have been sitting in that decanter for months instead of hours, and you can start to appreciate the danger.

Almost all crystal decanters sold in California now carry labels warning you not to use them to store liquids, especially alcohols. One manufacturer, Baccarat, has found a way to prevent lead leaching from its crystal. A fine film of lead-free glass is applied to the inside of the crystal, sealing the lead in and forming a barrier between the lead and the crystal's liquid contents. Other manufacturers are experimenting with processes that preleach lead from the surface of the crystal, in theory reducing the amount of lead available to cause contamination. California is taking a wait-and-see attitude on experimentation, until the companies can prove that preleaching is good for the long term.

By all means, bring the crystal out for special occasions. Decanting your sherry or brandy for an impressive evening is OK, too. Just remember to return what's left to the original bottle when the last guest has gone home.

By the way, if you've recently visited Wilshire Boulevard and plunked down $1,500 for a Steuben leaded-crystal decanter, don't be fooled by the lack of a California warning sticker. Steuben convinced the state that its decanters are meant to hold admiring gazes, not liqueurs. The Steuben decanters come with their own warning, telling customers to never, ever put anything alcoholic in them—the alcohol will etch the crystal and leave it cloudy. (Maybe the incredible clarity of Steuben crystal has something to do with the optical instrument glass I mentioned earlier.)

TIN CANS

We changed baby-sitters when Matthew was eighteen months old. One of his favorite foods at the time was minestrone soup. We'd open the can, drain the broth, and heat the pasta and vegetables. This horrified our new sitter; not the food, but the fact it came from a can. She's from Trinidad, and she told us she never uses canned food because it contains lead.

A tin can is a wonderfully simple thing, a piece of metal rolled into a cylinder, soldered, and capped. The problem is the solder. Common soft-solder, traditionally used to make the cans, is a lead-tin alloy containing as much as 98 percent lead. Fill the can with food, sit it on the shelf for a couple of months, and the leaching lead creates a poisonous potion.

As recently as the mid-1980s, the greatest exposure to lead for most people was the food they ate. Almost 50 percent of that lead came from the solder holding the tin can together. As late as 1990, it was estimated that 90 percent of all canned foods sold in the United States was packaged in lead-soldered cans. The food industry, under pressure from the FDA, voluntarily began to phase out the use of lead-soldered cans in 1991. Significantly, the baby food industry switched from tin cans to glass bottles, and almost overnight, the lead content in infant food dropped almost 90 percent. Unfortunately, the voluntary ban on soldered cans did not extend to imported foods, and though most western European countries ended the use of lead solder, other countries did not.

In mid-1993, while noting the Jumex fruit juice recall discussed at the beginning of the chapter, FDA Commissioner David A. Kessler estimated that some 10 percent of imported foods and beverages were still coming into the country in lead-soldered cans. He then moved to extend the ban, and in August 1994 it became illegal to import or sell lead-soldered cans containing products destined for consumption in the United States.

If you have any doubt about the safety of imported canned goods that may have been on the shelf for a prolonged period, look at the can seam before using the contents. Welded seams, the safe ones, are flat and smooth; soldered seams are raised, sometimes lumpy, with visible gray metal.

Protecting canned goods from lead contamination is especially important considering that canned foods are often significantly less expensive than foods packaged in other ways. They provide a major source of nutrition for the children of low-income families whose parents may already be dealing with other environmental lead threats.

WINE

Bottles of wine, both fine and table, have been wearing caps of soft lead foil for years. The tradition is a throwback to the days when the necks of newly bottled wine were dipped in hot wax to seal the cork. You may have noticed, after peeling the foil off, that a whitish powder was left on the rim of the bottle. The powdery deposit is lead salt that leached out of the foil. If it's not removed, it will dissolve readily into the wine as you pour.

The lead foil is disappearing, banished first by a number of key wine-producing states and now by the FDA. As a result, most wine corks are now sealed with a thin plastic cap, which looks much like its lead predecessor, or with recyclable aluminum. New York State, a major wine producer and consumer, was the leader in this effort, with a 1991 law limiting the level of lead in packaging to less than 100 ppm, so low it affects even the inks used to print wine labels. California dealt with lead foils under its Proposition 65 law. A number of major vintners there were sued and agreed in court to discontinue the use of lead caps and to produce a public education campaign informing people about how to deal with vintage wines capped with lead. Other wineries entered into the settlement to avoid being sued as well.

The federal regulation, covering both domestic and imported wines, was implemented in mid-1994 and in effect extended the ban to the vineyards that were bottling for local distribution in states without regulation. The FDA regulations, recognizing the unique nature and value of vintage wines, exempted wines bottled before the ban. Even without the federal ban, most wine bottled after 1991 will come without a lead cap. Vintage wine bottled before 1991 will most likely be capped with lead. Lead caps, however, are slowly passing into history. If you encounter one, wipe the cork and bottle top with a damp cloth until the white powder is removed.

CALCIUM SUPPLEMENTS

Next time you're in your local health-food store, read the labels on the calcium supplements: "No salt. No starch. No sugar. No preservatives.

No artificial color. No additives." The list goes on and on, sounding oh, so healthy. Unfortunately, the labels do not say "No lead."

It is ironic that in the pursuit of good health and nutrition, we might be poisoning ourselves and our children. That seems to be just the case with certain calcium supplements, often given to children who can't ingest milk products and frequently recommended to pregnant women and nursing mothers. They contain lead. Some contain a lot of lead.

We know all this because a Canadian scientist's son was allergic to milk. Dr. Bernard Bourgoin, a toxicologist with Environment Canada, the Canadian EPA, happened to do his doctoral research on the levels of lead found in the shells of mussels. When he was told to give his son a calcium supplement made from natural oyster shells, Dr. Bourgoin had second thoughts, reasoning that if mussel shells contained lead, oyster shells would too.

Dr. Bourgoin and his colleagues at Trent University in Ontario eventually tested 70 brands of calcium supplements. Most of them came from American suppliers or were sold in the United States. For 25 percent of the supplements tested, the suggested daily dose for children exceeded the maximum amount of lead that children six years and under are supposed to get from *all* dietary sources—in some cases by 200 to 400 percent.

The supplements tested were broken into five different categories, depending on the type and source of calcium. They were calcium phosphate or bonemeal, dolomite, calcium chelates, laboratory-refined calcium carbonate, and "natural source" calcium carbonate, mined from limestone rock composed of fossilized oyster shells. Most of the offending lead-laced calcium came from bonemeal and oyster shells, both natural sources.

By contrast, the calcium supplements lowest in lead were the refined calcium carbonates, which are laboratory processed. Every brand of this type of supplement tested at less than half the daily maximum. Refined calcium supplements start out natural, but the calcium is dissolved out of the natural source, then filtered and purified before being offered for sale.

How significant is the threat? According to government statistics, 8 percent of all children between the ages of two and six in the United States take an over-the-counter calcium supplement. So does one out of every four women, though there's no statistics telling how many may be pregnant or nursing. And there is evidence that low-income pregnant women, worried about poor diet, may double or even triple their recommended daily dose of calcium. There's the common misconception that if a little of something is good, a lot of it must be even better.

It's important to keep in mind that the ceiling of daily lead intake was not set at 6 μg (for children) because that figure is considered "safe." No level of lead is normal or safe; the daily maximum was set at this level because that is the lowest practical limit possible today. There is so much lead pollution in the environment that kids will accumulate 6 μg of lead every day simply by eating, drinking, and breathing. By extension, it's clear that to be safe, the lead level in calcium supplements must not exceed the lead level in milk, since the supplements are a substitution for milk, and milk is factored into the daily calculation.

Many calcium supplements, however, carry far more lead than does milk, and that excess lead is going to be on top of what's unavoidably consumed, and therefore on top of the recommended daily maximum. A lead content of 1 or 2 μg, such as found in the laboratory-processed calcium supplements, does not tilt the scales. Some supplements, however, contain so much lead that a daily dose would be enough to push a toddler over the CDC's 10 μg/dl action level, the point where both development and growth can be retarded. This should be a major concern.

Calcium supplements became a very real concern for health officials in Westchester County, New York. A case of childhood lead poisoning was referred to them for investigation. The caseworker who went to the child's house found both lead paint and a bottle of oyster shell calcium tablets. The mother said she was taking the tablets but had given them to her child on several occasions. Health officials tested the tablets and found they contained 12 ppm lead, equal to 12 μg/dl.

The FDA classifies vitamins and supplements as food, and therefore not subject to the higher standards of safety and effectiveness required of drugs. Dr. Michael Bolger, chief of the Contaminants Branch of the FDA, says the health risk of lead in calcium is not significant "in the grand scheme of things," referring to the risk posed by lead from paint and other sources, but quickly hastens to say that the FDA issued an advisory in 1982 cautioning against excess use of bonemeal and dolomite supplements and has been attempting to develop regulations for several years.

The effort has run into a classic bureaucratic snarl. Some calciums are used as food additives—turning up in all those "calcium fortified" products we see on the grocery shelf. Those additives fall into a category known in government acronymeze as GRAS, Generally Recognized As Safe. The GRAS safety decisions were made years ago, long before there was awareness of the danger posed by low-level lead, but they're in place, and calcium supplements can't be regulated without changing the GRAS list, and . . . well, you get the picture. It's going to be a while.

Though the risk from calcium supplements may be insignificant relative to the risk from lead-paint dust, it shouldn't be ignored. That would be like saying it's not important to keep kids from playing with matches since so many get hit by cars. Both risks need to be addressed. Dr. John Rosen, head of the lead program at the Montefiore Medical Center in the Bronx, New York, calls the situation "totally indefensible."

"There is no margin of safety for kids," he says, "given the overwhelming exposure to lead in the environment. To introduce new lead into a child's environment is totally unacceptable. The fact remains that this is a preventable source."

The presence of high levels of lead in calcium supplements is especially warped given that calcium (along with iron) is one of the two major dietary elements in combatting lead poisoning. Parents whose children have tested above the 10 µg/dl threshold are told to increase the calcium and iron contents of their child's diet and are often directed to use calcium supplements.

Industry, says one of Dr. Bourgoin's associates, needs to develop information on lead content in calcium and make it available to the consumer. Dr. Alfredo Quattrone, a California toxicologist who coauthored Dr. Bourgoin's study, says their work demonstrates that it's possible for all five basic types of calcium supplement to strictly limit lead content. Industry, he says, should move on a voluntary basis to eliminate lead from its product.

All of this is not to say you shouldn't take a calcium supplement if your doctor says that you or your child need to. Low-lead or lead-free calcium is available. Dr. Rosen recommends getting your calcium supplement through a prescription, since products manufactured for prescription are generally manufactured to a higher standard of purity.

The safest over-the-counter source of calcium is antacids. Because they claim to treat something (acid indigestion), they must meet the more stringent drug standards for purity and lack of toxicity. The two leading brands—Tums and Rolaids—are refined calcium carbonate.

Short of chowing down antacid, you should look for a calcium supplement that meets the standards of the United States Pharmacopeia (USP). Though it's not an absolute guarantee of purity— manufacturers displaying the USP symbol agree to meet the standards, but there is no testing or certification—the USP symbol is generally a dependable guideline. The USP level for lead in calcium is set at 3 ppm.

If you're looking for your supplement in a health-food store, shop in one that belongs to the National Nutritional Foods Association. Ask for a calcium supplement manufactured to association standards, which, like USP standards, are 3 ppm for lead in calcium.

As an extra caution, once you've selected your brand of supplement, write to the manufacturer and ask for a letter specifying the maximum levels of lead in this product. If the company isn't forthcoming, change brands.

BRASS AND BRONZE

Remember studying about the Bronze Age? That was when humans discovered that by melting and mixing naturally occurring metals, they could create new metals that were stronger, prettier, more easily worked or more resistant to rusting and corrosion. These metal mixtures are called alloys, and there are hundreds of them. Bronze and brass, originally made by mixing zinc or tin with copper, were among the first alloys created, and the golden luster of brass continues to bring warmth and beauty into our homes.

As we became more sophisticated, we added other metals, including lead, to the mix. Today, there are dozens of brass and bronze alloys, and many include lead. Brass objects found in the home typically contain about 3 percent lead and pose no threat whatsoever as long as you avoid certain food uses. (Others, like leaded bronze, not usually found in the home, contain up to 29 percent lead.) Items like brass candlesticks are completely harmless (unless your little one knocks them over and gets hit on the head, but that's a whole different scenario).

Brass bowls and plates and pitchers are fine for displaying flowers and nuts and solid fruits, but they shouldn't be used to serve or store liquids or wet or acidic foods. Setting out a brass bowl of chips or nuts for your party is fine; heating fondue or chili in a brass chafing dish is not. Likewise, don't serve tomato juice in a brass pitcher or hot mulled cider from a brass bowl. The reason is that acidic liquids, like fruit and vegetable juices, will leach the lead out of brass and bronze. Even a soft peach, sitting in a brass bowl, can soak up lead. Heating speeds the process, which is why you rarely see brass cookware or utensils.

PEWTER

Pewter is a soft malleable alloy made of tin and lead. It was in common use in Europe since the Roman times, and England, with its abundant quantities of tin, was Europe's pewter center since the Middle Ages. Pewter was Colonial America's chief tableware until it was displaced by china in the eighteenth century, and it's likely the first Thanksgiving meal was served on pewter. Paul Revere is known to have crafted pewter pieces. American colonists ate from pewter plates and porringers with pewter spoons and forks and quaffed their drinks from pewter tankards.

They undoubtedly paid a price. Pewter's lead content leaches readily. Early American pewterware belongs in museums, not on your table.

Modern pewter reproductions are made of a pewterlike metal technically called "Britannia." It's an alloy made of 93 percent tin, 6 percent antimony, and 1 percent copper. As you can see, it's totally lead-free and completely safe for serving food.

SILVER PLATE

Silver plate cups and bowls and platters are, by definition, a thin layer of silver or some other metal. The other metal is often an alloy containing lead. Unless you know that the silver plate is lead-free, use it as you would use a brass container. If your baby was given a silver plate baby cup, save it for ceremonial meals, and don't let acidic juices sit in it for any length of time. *Never store food or drink in a silver plate container.*

BREAD BAGS, ET CETERA

Colored inks contain lead. The plastic or cellophane bags that food is sold in are often printed with bright-colored lead-tint inks. The food inside is perfectly safe, since the ink is on the outside. However, the bags shouldn't be reused to store food; elevated lead levels have been found in food that was stored in bread wrappers that had been turned inside out.

For the same reason, while it's okay to wrap a fish in the *New York Times,* don't use *USA Today* or the Sunday funnies!

8

OUTSIDE YOUR HOME

*None of the child care agencies in the
16 states we contacted had compiled
data on the results of lead inspections
at child care facilities.*

—*U.S. General Accounting Office
"Report to Congress" (September 1993)*

MOST KIDS HAVE TROUBLE getting their parents interested in their science fair project, but not thirteen-year-old Nichole Connolly of the West Iredell Middle School in Statesville, North Carolina. She even was able to get ABC's "Good Morning America" interested in hers.

The seventh-grader's project started out simply enough. She had read about lead poisoning and proposed testing drinking water in local schools. Her science teacher knew that the schools were on a municipal water system with stringent water standards but agreed nonetheless; the point of a science fair project, after all, is to learn the process, not to make some startling discovery.

So Nichole went to a local laboratory and arranged to have someone mentor her as she tested for lead. Then she went to the schools. She'd done her homework and asked to be shown a faucet that wasn't used very often. She carefully took and labeled "first draw" and flushed-system samples and headed to the lab. From each sample, she measured exactly 100 ml of water into a container, added nitric acid, and then tested the results on an AA/AE spectrophotometer, a professional instrument for measuring lead levels. A computer did the calculations and spit out a report card. One school flunked.

Nichole's sample from the Pressly Elementary School came from a faucet in the art room. It tested 17.7 ppb, over the EPA limit of 15 ppb and well above average levels for local water. Nichole didn't believe her eyes; she went back to the school, drew a new sample, and retested. Still above 17; her science project was a success beyond anyone's expectations.

School officials immediately tested all the faucets in the Pressly School. All were normal. Except the faucet in the art room. Tests showed the faucet itself to be the source of the lead. It has since been replaced. And Nichole Connolly won first place in her division at the science fair.

While Nichole was talking about her project on ABC's "Good Morning America," a TV station in Washington, D.C., was taking water samples in schools in the nation's capital. Reporters from WJLA-TV discovered high levels of lead coming from water fountains in several schools. What's worse, the station checked school records and learned that school officials had previously tested the water fountains and knew they were hazardous. A fountain at one school tested 76 times the allowable limit yet was still bubbling away. School administrators had no explanation.

These incidents illustrate how the risk of childhood lead poisoning extends beyond the home. Schools, churches, and community centers have plumbing systems that are as likely to contain lead as your home is, and many of these buildings have lead paint on their walls. We've already talked about how the exhaust from cars and trucks and emissions from industry have polluted soil everywhere. As a parent, you need to take everything you've learned about looking for lead in your home and apply it to every place your child spends any time.

CHECKING FOR HAZARDS: YOU MUST DO IT YOURSELF

The more time your child spends in a given location, the more thorough your evaluation needs to be. We took a long, hard look at the day-care center where Matthew spends three full days a week but took just a cursory glance at his grandmother's home, where he spends a couple of nights a month. Be prudent, but be sensible.

Remember that leaded paint—in old buildings, on old woodwork and furniture, and on the ground outside—represents the greatest risk. At the grandparents', look out for an antique crib or toys, brought down from the attic. In the church nursery, check the paint on window-sills and dust in window wells. In the playground, look for nearby buildings or structures that might have shed peeling lead paint. Most neighborhood parents, if they're smart, end up taking turns watching each other's children. Make sure your neighbor's house isn't in the midst of renovation work if your child is going to spend time there.

If your child is like most today, she will spend at least some time in day care or preschool. With the increase in single-parent homes and families where both parents work, many infants and toddlers spend more waking hours in day care than they do at home. The government estimates that 4.5 million children are in registered child-care facilities and doesn't even hazard a guess at how many more are in unregulated day-care situations. You must make certain they are in a safe environment, and you must do it yourself. One of America's great lapses in dealing with lead poisoning is the failure to require that day-care centers, preschools, and schools be lead-free.

In September 1993, the GAO issued a report to the House Subcommittee on Health and the Environment titled "The Extent of Lead Hazards in Child Care Facilities Is Unknown." The GAO report said that although several federal agencies have programs dealing with lead in general, few of the programs address lead in child-care facilities and schools, and those few programs that do are applied to only a narrow selection of special situations. No one at any level of government, federal or state, has collected information on the extent to which child-care facilities and schools contain lead hazards. There is not even a uniform requirement that they be tested, and few districts, the GAO learned, test for lead in paint, universally recognized as posing the greatest risk.

While *all* schools certainly should be free of lead, remember that your child is at greatest risk in her earliest years; the potential for lead poisoning falls off significantly about the time she turns seven. Lead exposure in preschools and day-care centers poses the greatest threat of childhood lead poisoning, and a parent's checklist should include questions about lead:

■ Check every space or room where your child will be spending time, including playing, eating, changing, and sleeping areas. Ask where food is prepared, and check there as well. Do the children play in the basement in bad weather? Take a look.

■ Look for peeling paint or signs that children have been chewing on paint. How clean are the floors, windowsills, and, especially, window wells? If the building is not new, ask if the paint has been tested for lead.

■ Ask if the water has been tested for lead. If so, ask to see the results. School drinking water should contain less than 20 ppb lead. Look to see if there's a water cooler (see next section and appendix J).

■ Do the children play outside? Check the yard or playground, looking for buildings or overhead structures that could be dropping lead-paint chips into the yard. How close is the play area to heavily traveled streets and roads? Has the soil been tested for lead? (These questions will be addressed later in this chapter.)

■ Check art supplies, especially chalk, crayons, and finger paints. If they are not made in the United States (and especially if they are made in China), they are suspect for containing poisonous levels of lead (see chapters 9 and 10).

While you need to be especially alert to the presence of lead when using family day care, since it is subject to the least regulation, the examples of Nichole Connolly and the reporter in Washington point up the fact that lead can lurk in even the most regulated atmosphere. If you find a potential problem, discuss it with whoever runs the school or facility. The seriousness of the situation and this individual's responsiveness to it should dictate whether you consider placing or keeping your child there. By no means, however, should you allow your child to go to—or stay in—a facility that has chipping, peeling paint or that is being renovated.

If you discover a serious problem and your child is already attending the facility, talk not only to the staff but also to other parents. This is a situation that demands that you become an activist! You owe it to other parents to make them aware of the risk to their children, and you may need their help in forcing action. Check, too, with your local health officials; some states and many cities do have programs dealing with lead in facilities that cater to young children. Ask if the care center or school has been inspected, and if it has, ask to see the record of the inspection. In New York City, the New York Public Interest Research Group recently charged that the city's health department had found paint with high levels of lead in 69 private and public preschools and had not notified the schools.

LEAD IN SCHOOL WATER COOLERS

Ironically, although the EPA says leaded paint is the greatest danger to young children in preschools or day-care centers, followed by lead in soil, the only source of exposure that has been addressed to date at the national level is lead in school drinking water. That's due in large part to the compelling testimony given before Congress by Paul Mushak, professor of environmental pathology at the University of North Carolina-Chapel Hill. Professor Mushak told of the high levels of lead delivered by water fountains in public schools. Many of the ubiquitous water coolers, he explained, contained lead-lined water storage tanks. Water sits in them—overnight, over the weekend, over breaks, even over the summer—until the amount of lead leached into the water reaches extraordinary levels. Because they have storage tanks, running the water to flush them isn't a practical solution.

The Congress was stirred into action and passed the Lead Contamination Control Act (LCCA). The states were told to set up programs to help schools and day-care centers test for lead. The EPA was ordered to compile a list of all water coolers containing lead and to publish information on how school officials could ensure a lead-free water supply. The Consumer Product Safety Commission (CPSC) was told to issue a recall of water coolers containing lead-lined storage tanks. That was in 1988.

In 1991, the Natural Resources Defense Council surveyed three territories and the 50 states to measure the law's effectiveness. Six states didn't know whether any schools had been tested, and another 16 reported less than a quarter of all schools tested. When it came to preschool or day care—the facilities dealing with the children at greatest risk—only 17 states had tested any. The total tested came to 0.6 percent of the nation's *licensed* child-care facilities, with no mention of the estimated one million unlicensed ones.

As to removing the lead-spouting water coolers, which involved simply comparing the make and model against the EPA list, only 19 states reported checking any schools, and only one locality, the territory of Guam, checked all the water coolers in all of its schools. Halsey Taylor, manufacturer of the coolers with lead-lined tanks, negotiated a Consent Order Agreement with the CPSC under which it agreed to replace or issue a refund for any unit made before April 1, 1979. Terms of the recall included many limitations, however, and the company reported replacing 514 of the lead-contaminated units by the end of 1990, with refund checks mailed for an additional 105 units. There is no public record of how many of these units may have been made and sold, so there is no way to judge the effectiveness of the CPSC-negotiated recall. However, an EPA news release issued in 1989 says Halsey Taylor, EBCO Manufacturing, and Sunroc Corporation had answered a congressional survey by estimating that almost one million water coolers containing lead had been made and were probably still in use.

There were lots of excuses. Congress passed the law but didn't give the states any money to carry it out. The EPA was a year late in issuing the list of lead-lined water coolers that needed to be removed. The law only urged schools to test their water. Neither testing nor reporting was made mandatory. In 1990, an internal audit by the inspector general's office criticized the EPA for the delay in publishing the list of dangerous water coolers and for failing to "aggressively locate and identify additional coolers to place on the list." The inspector general's report said that while many schools discovered dangerous levels of lead in their drinking water, many other schools "did not test their water, and if they did test, they did not always test adequately." School administrators blamed "confusing" federal requirements.

The inspector general's audit called on both the EPA and the states to become more aggressive in eliminating the health hazard posed by lead in drinking water. One of the schools where WJLA reporters found lead-lined water coolers still in use some three and a half years after the IG's report is located less than five miles from EPA headquarters in Washington!

So it's up to you as a parent to become an investigative reporter. Start by taking the list of water coolers known to contain lead (see appendix J) to your school or day-care center and looking at the manufacturer's label. If you find one that's on the list, it should be shut off immediately. If there's a question, take a water sample, preferably early on a Monday morning, and get it tested. And if you don't get immediate action, call your local TV station! When WJLA aired its reports in Washington, the Young Elementary School officials fell over themselves to shut off the offending water fountains.

People responsible for safety of children's drinking water, ranging from school officials and school board members to local activists and parents involved in co-op day care, should get a copy of the EPA booklet "Lead in School Drinking Water." It was published as part of the LCAA mandate and is an excellent source of information on everything from testing faucets, fountains, and ice machines to the larger responsibilities of schools that supply their own water from wells. The booklet is available for $3.25 from: The Superintendent of Documents, U.S.

Government Printing Office, Washington, DC 20402, GPO Stock Number 055-000-00281-9. You may be able to get a free copy by asking your local congressman.

LEAD PAINT IN SCHOOLS AND DAY-CARE CENTERS

If attitudes about lead in water coolers have been this blasé, even in the face of national legislation and EPA outreach, you can imagine what's being done about lead in paint—prevalent in schools and day-care centers, potentially expensive and difficult to address, and ignored by most lawmakers.

Although lead paint is universally recognized as the primary source of childhood lead exposure, the 1993 GAO investigation commissioned by the House Health and Environment Subcommittee found that little or nothing was being done about it. The comptroller general surveyed 16 states and found:

■ Almost half (seven) of these states conduct no inspections of child-care facilities for lead hazards.

■ Only two routinely inspect any child-care facilities for lead paint. (Only one inspects for lead-contaminated soil.)

■ Out of 57 school districts examined by the GAO, only nine inspect any schools for lead paint. (Only three inspect for lead-contaminated soil.)

The GAO report concludes: "*Many child-care facilities and schools are taking little or no action to protect children from lead hazards in paint and soil*" (original emphasis).

There isn't even a data base to tell us how big the problem is. We can guess: The vast majority of schools in the United States, especially in urban centers, were built before the ban on leaded paint. New York City, which banned the use of lead paint in residential work in 1960, was still using lead-based industrial paint on its schools in 1980, and that covers 97 percent of the classrooms in use today.

We should expect to find significant lead-paint problems in day-care centers too. They work on tight budgets and are usually located in older, often poorly maintained, buildings. The GAO investigators did find one valuable source of information on lead exposure in child-care facilities, and the news was not good. South Carolina spent six years inspecting more than 3,200 child-care and foster-home facilities; the state found that almost 20 percent had lead hazards. At one child-care center, in Charleston, more than 40 percent of the enrolled children had toxic levels of lead in their blood.

Preschools and day-care centers, which house children at their age of greatest risk, should be our top priority. They should be the first tested, and they should be at the head of the line for remedial money and action. They're not. Child-care centers are often stand-alone operations. A few are cooperatively run; some are business ventures; many are nonprofit; each has its own governing body. It's simply easier to go after school systems, where there's a central board and administration that can be pressured.

In New York City, a coalition of angry parents forced the school chancellor to appoint a task force to recommend reductions of lead hazards in the city schools. The House subcommittee that was investigating the extent of school lead exposure took the report of the chancellor's task force and applied it to New York City Board of Education maintenance records showing the level of classroom paint damage. The subcommittee determined that one classroom in six in New York had a lead hazard. Unfortunately, the task force decided that intact lead paint was not an immediate lead hazard and that only damaged lead paint qualified for abatement. This decision totally ignored the risk posed by the lead dust generated by the daily opening and closing of heavily painted doors and drawers and windows and cabinets in pre-K, kindergarten, and first-grade classrooms—classrooms housing the children at greatest risk.

Failure to recognize that *children of different ages face different risks* becomes apparent again when the report of the House subcommittee investigation lists "The Twelve Most Hazardous Schools." Four of them are high schools! The city will be forced to expend its very limited resources to abate peeling paint in high schools before it ensures that floors and windowsills in entry-level classrooms are properly cleaned to limit lead dust, and long before it gets around to lead-paint testing in day-care centers and preschools.

OTHER SOURCES OF LEAD EXPOSURE

You may need to learn some local history to adequately protect your child from other sources of lead exposure. Schools and parks and playgrounds are often built next to or even on top of everything from former industrial sites to municipal landfills. If contamination connected with the sites were cleaned up and the landfills properly capped, there should be no problem, but that is too seldom the case. Start by asking the Board of Education or the Parks Department about your area. Ask your local Board of Health. Talk to some old-timers or the local newspaper. You can also file a Freedom of Information Act (FOIA) request with your regional office of the EPA. A sample FOIA letter is included in appendix K and a list of regional EPA offices is included in appendix F. If a historical search turns up a potential source of contamination, ask to see the results of testing done to determine risk. If tests weren't done in the past, they should be done now.

Some sources of lead contamination can be found just by looking around. We talked in chapter 5 about neighborhoods contaminated by lead paint flaking off steel bridges. The rain of toxic paint does not fall just on homes. The Williamsburg Bridge sandblasting dumped lead concentrations of 17,856 ppm in an outdoor basketball court and a staggering 46,092 ppm in a local playground. No child should be exposed to these levels, however briefly.

The Williamsburg experience led other bridge operators in New York to examine the land within their shadow: the Triborough Bridge Authority, which operates a number of major bridges, told parents to keep children from playing in several playgrounds until their safety could be assured. The City Parks Department eventually closed sections of five parks, including city baseball fields across the street from Yankee Stadium, until parks workers could sweep and vacuum up the toxic chips that littered the play areas.

If your child plays in an area under or near an overhead bridge, highway, water tower, or other steel structure that could be the source of lead paint, ask if the soil has been tested. Better yet, get a sample tested yourself. In the meantime, don't send food to the playground, and make sure your child washes up before eating.

Parents in Cortland, New York, didn't have to look to find the source of lead pollution in their neighborhood; they could hear it. Cortland is home to the beautiful 1,800-acre Blue Mountain Reservation, filled with walking paths and hiking trails. And the county-operated shooting range. The Westchester County Sportsmen's Center opened for business in 1962. Since then, an estimated 300 tons of lead have been shot into the environment, one bullet at a time. Inevitably, the lead-contaminated soil began to wash away, until it ultimately polluted Furnace Brook, which runs through the reservation and then past the Furnace Woods Elementary School. A fence was built between the school playground and the brook to keep children from playing in the lead-contaminated water. The school also installed an outdoor sink so children could wash their hands before entering the school building.

The situation eventually wound up in the regional office of the EPA, which took action under a section of the Resource Conservation and Recovery Act (RCRA). The EPA's authority to act was upheld, and in 1994 the county of Westchester agreed to remediate the lead contamination and ensure there will be no future recontamination. The case set an important precedent, but it's by no means the first time that lead pollution from a shooting range has threatened a community. After the city of Chicago evicted a gun club from its shooting range on the shores of Lake Michigan, the city had to remove some 8,000 cubic yards of lead-contaminated soil, and similar situations may exist at as many as 8,000 public and private shooting ranges.

While it took federal action to get the Westchester Sportsmen Center site cleaned up, it was parental action that started the ball moving. And so it is with most lead prevention and remediation activities. You simply cannot rely on governmental bodies to protect your child from the silent threat of lead poisoning.

9

OCCUPATIONS AND HOBBIES

Childhood lead poisoning is a man-made disease.

—*Herbert L. Needleman, M.D.*

THE SPANISH ARTIST Francisco de Goya moved from the gentle rococo style of *The Picnic* to the dark, nightmarish images of his final *Los proverbios*. Was this the natural evolution of an artist tortured by the horror of war, or the tormented result of poisoning from a lifetime working with leaded pigments? No one knows for certain, but Goya suffered recurrent illnesses characterized by impaired speech, vision, and hearing, and later by partial paralysis, all evidence of lead poisoning.

People work with lead. On the job, in their profession, and at home, pursuing their hobbies. People who work with lead professionally bring it into their homes by accident; people who use lead recreationally bring it into the home in shopping bags and UPS parcels. Few of them are fully aware of what they're doing.

OCCUPATIONAL LEAD POISONING

This type of lead poisoning has been described in medical literature since the writings of Hippocrates himself. It seems so obvious, but people often overlook the lead dust they pick up on the job as a potential source of exposure for their children. Lead dust clings to people's skin and hair. It gets under workers' fingernails. It becomes enmeshed in the fabric of their clothing, and it sticks to their shoes. It can travel home in their lunchpails and on their vehicles.

A Memphis, Tennessee, study in the 1970s of children of lead-industry workers found that more than 40 percent of them had blood-lead levels in excess of 30 μg/dl; 10 percent of them were suffering Class V lead poisoning, with lead levels above 80 μg/dl. The children's blood-lead levels correlated directly with the concentration of lead in dust samples taken from the families' homes. A study of the lead content in carpeting in the homes of battery workers found levels ranging from 1,700 ppm to 84,050 ppm in children's bedrooms. In Colorado, a young man who ground cast-lead buckles smooth was hospitalized with acute lead poisoning and treated with chelation. Health officials found he had brought so much lead dust home in his clothing that his wife and three daughters also required chelation treatment, and his youngest daughter eventually needed retreatment.

Strict compliance with the Occupational Safety and Health Administration (OSHA) lead standard, adopted in 1978, protects against this exposure, but many workers are not covered by the OSHA umbrella. So-called cottage industries, companies with fewer than 10 employees, are exempt from OSHA regulation. Small "craft" pottery studios and stained-glass ateliers, both of which work with lead, are often small enough to escape mandatory worker protection.

OSHA's General Industry Lead Standard was both enlightened and precedent setting when adopted. It requires employers to provide safety information and training for workers who use lead, and to monitor the level of lead not only in the workplace air but also in the worker's blood. The law protects workers' jobs as well as their health, requiring that the employer preserve a worker's job, wages, and seniority if the employee has to stop work because of elevated blood-lead levels. Workers are removed from the job if their blood-lead level exceeds 50 μg/dl; they cannot return until it drops below 40 μg/dl.

Several studies show, however, that compliance with OSHA lead standards is inadequate; in 1987, more than 200 lead-industry workers in New York, New Jersey, and California were found to have blood-lead levels above 50 μg/dl. Additionally, in the time since the standards were written, toxic effects have been proven at levels far below the 40 and 50 μg/dl triggers, and the CDC now says that current OSHA standards for lead may not adequately protect the health of workers.

Pregnant women working in the lead industry are of special concern. Lead crosses the placenta, and a pregnant woman's blood-lead level becomes her fetus's blood-lead level. Lead exposure also increases the incidence of spontaneous abortion. Instead of reducing workplace lead pollution to prevent this exposure, many segments of the industry have adopted exclusionary policies. These "fetal protection policies" prevent pregnant women—and in some cases all fertile women—from holding jobs working with lead.

Ironically, construction workers—including demolition and lead-abatement workers—are not covered by OSHA's General Industry Lead Standard. Although these workers are at particularly high risk of having very high blood-lead levels, they are covered under a much weaker standard. Pliny advised that lead miners in the Roman Empire protect themselves against lead by wearing an animal bladder tied tightly across the face, yet you can drive up any street today and see workmen sanding lead-based paint without so much as a dust mask.

OSHA is currently working with the National Institute for Occupational Safety and Health (NIOSH) to review health data relating to construction workers and intends to issue a revised lead-in-construction standard. The state of Maryland decided not to wait; it enacted more stringent lead-worker and construction-worker safety standards.

The occupations that expose workers to lead are obvious and well known (see list), but there are still hidden hazards. The CDC recently issued a warning to electricians after a Columbus, Ohio, electrical worker's lead poisoning was traced to his habit of chewing the plastic coating stripped from wires. Kenneth Galbraith's symptoms included tingling in his fingers, mild memory loss, and diminished math skills. He was tested for lead poisoning, and his blood-lead level was more than ten times the norm. His family tested normal, and health investigators were stumped until he mentioned his nervous habit of chewing plastic insulation. Lead is used in the manufacture of plastic and in the pigments used to color it; the insulation tested off the scale.

INDUSTRIES, OCCUPATIONS, AND PRODUCTS INVOLVING WORK WITH LEAD

Ammunition manufacture
Auto body refinishing
Auto parts and accessories
Auto radiator repair shops
Auto repairers
Automotive repair shops

Boatyard workers
Brass/copper foundry
Bridge, tunnel, and elevated-highway construction
Cable makers, splicers
Chemicals and chemical preparations
Construction workers
Demolition workers
Firing-range workers
Fishing-sinker manufacturers
Gas stations
Glass manufacturers
Industrial machinery and equipment
Inorganic pigments manufacturers
Jewelers
Lead-abatement workers
Lead miners
Lead smelters and refiners
Metal polishers
Painters
Plastic manufacturers
Plumbers/pipe fitters
Plumbing-fixture fittings and trim manufacturers
Police officers
Pottery and ceramics
Primary batteries, dry and wet
Printers
Recycling facilities
Roofers
Rubber-product manufacturers
Scrap, sheet metal workers
Sculptors using solder
Secondary smelting and refining of nonferrous metals
Shellac makers
Shipbuilders
Shipyard workers
Stained-glass makers
Steel welders/cutters
Storage batteries (lead batteries)
Textile makers
Valve and pipe-fittings manufacturers
Welders

THE RISKS CONNECTED WITH ARTS AND CRAFTS

One person's profession may be another's hobby. It is in the field of arts and crafts that the line between vocation and avocation blurs. The same materials are used by all. The studio may be in a separate factory building or loft, or it can be in a spare bedroom or even a corner of the living room. Ceramics, stained glass, jewelry, metal sculpture, enameling, printing, and painting all may involve the use of lead in some form or another.

Judy Katz's* pottery studio was the back half of the 600-foot loft that doubled as her family's home. The two areas were separated by a corridor and a plastic curtain. She frequently airbrushed fritted-lead glazes (discussed in detail later in this section) onto ceramic tiles. She wore an OSHA-approved respirator but worked without ventilation. As her daughter got older, she spent more time in the studio with her mother, starting to paint and glaze her own pottery. Judy fitted a paper mask over her daughter's face.

Judy reported beginning to feel fatigue but ascribed that to the long days of a working mother. She also had occasional bouts of dizziness, and when a new label on one of her glaze products described potential lead hazards, Judy went for a blood test. Her lead level was 48 μg/dl; her five-year-old daughter was then tested and showed a 54 μg/dl level. It was months after the elimination of lead-containing compounds before the little girl's blood-lead levels came within acceptable limits. But the lead collected in 17 years of exposure had been stored in Judy's bones, and nearly two years after her initial visit to the doctor, Judy's lead level was still above 20 μg/dl.

At the nonprofit Center for Safety in the Arts (CSA) in New York City, there's one entire file drawer filled with case histories of artists and artisans, professionals and hobbyists, adults and children, all unknowingly poisoned while working with lead. The center receives, on average, two calls a week from people whose work history and/or symptoms would indicate lead poisoning. Those suspicions are frequently borne out by subsequent blood-lead testing. Cases include:

- A woman jeweler who worked at home and whose blood-lead level was 56 μg/dl.

*In order to protect individual's privacy, real name has been changed.

■ Two stained-glass artists whose blood-lead levels were 42 and 48 μg/dl.

■ Two enamelists whose blood-lead levels were 53 and 83 μg/dl.

■ A glaze mixer at a small pottery studio whose blood-lead level was 80 μg/dl after only four months on the job.

■ A Jewish scribe hospitalized with grand mal seizure whose blood-lead level was 136 μg/dl. The scribe wrote holy scripture on parchment with a feather pen, frequently licking the pen to maintain a fine point. The traditional ink he used was found to be 13,000 ppm lead.

Old ways die hard, and artists persist in using lead even when safer products are readily available. Some painters still prime their canvas with flake white or white lead primer, avowing that it's more durable than other whites. A salesman for Lee's Art Shops, a large chain in New York City, says that despite the dangers and difficulties of working with white lead primer—it takes forever to dry—his store still sells quite a lot. Monona Rossol, contributing editor of *Art Hazard News*, wrote in November 1981 about some of the many ways in which artists, craftspeople, and hobbyists are exposed to lead:

■ Painting: painting, spraying, or airbrushing lead-containing oils, acrylics, automobile paints, boat paints, or metal rust-inhibiting paints; grinding pigments; sanding paints or gesso; heating paints with torches; tipping brushes with the lips.

■ Ceramics: working with lead glazes, lustres, frits, or lead-containing glaze chemicals; inhaling kiln fumes; eating from improperly glazed dinnerware.

■ Metal casting: casting lead-containing bronzes or other lead-alloyed metals; finishing, chasing, or applying patinas to these metals.

■ Lead casting: making bullets, lead soldiers, cast- and dripped-lead sculpture.

■ Pewter work: casting of old-formula (lead-containing) pewter; soldering, finishing, and sanding pewter.

■ Stained glass: handling, soldering (both the regular and the copper foil method), sanding, applying patinas to lead came (stained glass is covered in more detail later in this section), and applying and firing glass enamels and paints.

■ Glassblowing: making and working with lead glass; using lead-containing colorants; applying glass enamels and paints; grinding and polishing lead glass.

■ Art conservation and antique restoration: repairing or removing old paint and gesso; torching old paint; working with many old lead-containing metals and materials.

■ Welding: inhaling lead fumes from welding lead-painted metals such as old car parts.

■ Printmaking: using inks colored with lead pigments.

■ Photography: using the platinum process which employs lead oxalate.

■ Rubber-mold making: when curing agent is lead peroxide.

■ Enameling: working with lead-frit enamels, inhaling kiln fumes.

Source: Center for Safety in the Arts "Lead Poisoning" Fact Sheet, November, 1981.

It goes almost without saying that if there are children in the home while you engage in any of these activities, they as well as you will be exposed. Children should be kept out of your studio or work area at all times, not just while you're working. Lead dust and residue remain long after your project is complete. Remember that children, especially at the toddler stage, will taste and eat almost anything. Keep leaded materials safely out of reach.

GLAZES AND FRITS

During 1991, the most recent year for which statistics are available, the American Association of Poison Control Centers reported 318 incidents of ceramic glaze ingestion. Although the thrust of this book deals with children, the dangers of using lead ceramic glaze in recreational therapy programs and nursing home programs must be noted: There are a number of reported incidents of accidental ingestion of lead glaze in nursing homes (resulting in at least one death) and deliberate ingestion by suicidal patients in occupational therapy situations.

Lead pottery glazes are the most common source of lead poisoning among artisans and hobbyists. This situation stems partly from misinformation, partly from poor procedures in the studio. Lead-bearing glaze is doubly dangerous, for it can poison the ceramic object's end user as well as the artist who made it. When WNBC television in New York tested handcrafted pottery items (brought in by staff members) for leaching lead, three of the six items tested leached high levels. Two of the pieces that failed were made by craftspeople. The third item was a ceramic cup made by a child at a local crafts program and brought home with all the pride associated with a child's handiwork. The child was exposed to lead not only during the crafting of the cup but every time she later drank from it.

Many art teachers still believe that some forms of lead are safe, that certain lead frits (frits are powders that are mixed with other ingredients to make a glaze) are nonsoluble and therefore safe to use. In fact, all lead frits are soluble to some degree; some are up to 50 percent soluble. This means that their lead contents will be released if they're ingested. In addition, lead fumes can escape from the kiln during firing and either be breathed in directly or settle out as a fine lead dust that is later ingested through children's normal hand-to-mouth activity. The lead fumes that don't escape the kiln condense on the surface of everything in the kiln, effectively contaminating every piece fired in the kiln, even those that started out with lead-free glazing.

Another problem stems from a misunderstanding of glaze labeling. The term *lead-safe* applied to glaze means that the finished product, if properly fired, will be safe to use for serving or storing food, meaning it won't leach lead. Even that claim is suspect, because the prevention of lead leaching requires careful attention to firing, often at temperatures and temperature control that's impossible to achieve in the small electric kilns typically found in homes and classrooms. That concern aside, "lead-safe" frits and glaze contain lead and are not safe for children to handle.

The only truly safe glazes and frits are those that carry the AP or CP seal of the Arts and Crafts Materials Institute; they are leadless or lead-free. AMACO, which is one of the largest suppliers of ceramics materials to schools, says its lead-free products clearly carry the AP seal as well as the word *lead-free*. AMACO says the trend, even among professionals, is toward lead-free products, and the company has worked to reformulate more and more lead-free products. However, the company warns teachers (and parents) to check labels to be sure they have the new lead-free product, not an old lead-bearing product that's been sitting on the stockroom shelf.

Home potters who insist on using lead glaze should test their end product for lead leaching if it can in any way be used for food serving or storage. One of the test kits listed in appendix I, marketed by Frandon Enterprises, was developed by Frances and Donald Wallace of Seattle after they became poisoned by lead leaching from Italian coffee cups. The Frandon kit was evaluated by the FDA and was found to be "capable of readily detecting lead levels of 2 ppm or more." Although this level of sensitivity is not enough to guarantee compliance with either FDA standards or the far more stringent California Prop. 65 standards (see chapter 7), the Frandon kit can be used as an inexpensive way to screen the effectiveness of your firing. Note that this kit releases a poisonous gas, hydrogen sulfide, and should be used either outdoors or in a ventilated area.

STAINED GLASS

Another artisan activity that frequently causes lead poisoning is stained-glass work. A letter in the CSA files from a Milwaukee stained-glass artist reads in part:

> I became so engrossed in my work, I turned on the soldering iron before breakfast—first things first, and had breakfast while fabricating, lunch too, and when things really got busy (Christmas orders), many times I worked fourteen hours a day in that contaminated air. No wonder I got so sick. I blamed the early symptoms of nausea and constant diarrhea on working too long.

Stained-glass artists heat, draw, bend, solder, grind, and polish the thin strips of grooved lead called *came* that separate and connect the individual pieces of colored glass. Artists breathe in both fumes and dust of the lead they work with. Their skin, hair, shoes, and clothing are contaminated with lead dust. Their hands carry it to their mouths, and their clothing carries it out of the studio. Studies have shown direct correlation between the amount of exposure—how often and how long they work—and the level of lead in the artist's blood.

Stained-glass work done in the home is, if anything, even more hazardous to children than is ceramic work. The fumes and dust are largely invisible and difficult to contain. It's hard to conceive of any safe way for an artist to work with lead came in a home that includes very young children.

It is possible to create lead-free stained glass, but the materials are more difficult to work with. Zinc came is available, but it's not as malleable as lead. Lead-free solders are also available (see next section).

SOLDER AND MOLTEN LEAD

Anyone working with solder—of any type—or with molten lead should heed the advice of a longtime salesman at the S. A. Bendheim Company in New York: "Don't boil the solder, and keep your fingers out of your mouth." Sculptors and jewelers who solder metal pieces, hobbyists who cast metal figures, plaques, or medallions, sportsmen who mold bullets or lead fishing sinkers—all put themselves and their children at risk. Artisans crafting jewelry should also avoid the use of cadmium-based solder. Cadmium in even tiny amounts is believed to cause cancer.

You might consider working with one of the lead-free solders. These solders come in either pewter or silver finish, and using one of them would certainly lessen your exposure. The complaints about lead-free solders have to do with flow and wetting action, so you may need to experiment to find one you're comfortable with.

Lead casting used to be a common childhood craft project for older children. Lead melts at a low temperature (620° F, hence its use in solder) and could be poured into little molds to create small figures and toys. Lead casting remains a home hobby for adults, sometimes as an end unto itself, casting medals and figurines, more often as part of an unrelated hobby. Sportsmen may cast lead to make their own bullets. Others cast their own fishing sinkers (now illegal). Long before I knew better, I collected used wheel weights from local garages and melted them down to cast a lead counterweight for a home-built telescope.

Obviously, kids under six shouldn't be around when you're doing this work. Aside from the danger from splatters and burns, there are two dangers that may result in lead poisoning. Heating lead releases lead fumes or vapors into the room. Minute particles of lead are then carried through the air, representing the most dangerous form of lead pollution since they are most readily absorbed by the body. (Melting and casting lead should be done only in a well-ventilated area, and you should wear an appropriate respirator while you're heating and pouring.) The other danger to children is posed by the little splatters that can end up on the floor. They are shiny-bright, certain to attract little eyes, and they're soft, malleable, and interesting to chew. They will certainly leave a lead residue on a child's fingers, and chances are only too good they'll end up in the child's stomach.

PRECAUTIONS TO TAKE WHEN WORKING WITH LEAD

If you work with lead, either professionally or as a craft or hobby, you should take the following precautions:

- Get frequent blood-lead tests. If you work at home, have your children's lead level tested as well.
- Use an exhaust ventilation system, where provided.
- Use the correct, clean respirator. Activities resulting in high lead exposure require the use of an air-purifying respirator with a NEPA filter.
- Keep the work area clean. Use only a HEPAvac or wet cleaning with a lead-binding solution for removing lead dust. Do not use compressed air to clear lead dust.
- Wash hands and face before eating, drinking, smoking, blowing your nose, applying cosmetics—or handling children.
- Eat, drink, and smoke in an area away from any lead. Keep lunch boxes, food, and coffee cups away from lead dust.
- Use protective clothing. Keep street clothes away from your work area.
- If possible, shower and change into clean clothes before leaving the work area. If you drive to lunch or elsewhere during the day, change before getting in the car so it doesn't become contaminated. Those who work off the premises should never wear contaminated work clothes, including shoes, home.
- Don't park where lead-dust from the job site can contaminate your vehicle.

Any hobby that may release lead into the home environment, either through heating or by sanding and grinding, must be pursued in a separate area of your home, and small children should be kept out. These activities should never be carried out in a corner of the kitchen. Don't even store or clean leaded material on the kitchen counter or in the sink; the danger of contaminating your child's food is just too great. Your work area should be kept clean, and off-limits to little people to prevent ingestion of dust through normal hand-to-mouth activities and to prevent accidental poisoning by your child's exploratory eating.

CHOOSE ART SUPPLIES CAREFULLY

Take the time to read the label before buying materials for use in your workshop or your crafts or artistic hobbies. Be especially careful to read the label on any art supplies you purchase for use by children. (See the section "Toys" in chapter 10.) In some cases, you may be able to completely eliminate the use of lead in your work. There are lead-free alternatives to everything from stained-glass solder to glaze and canvas gesso.

A new law, the Labeling of Hazardous Art Materials Act, went into effect in November 1990. The law takes what had been a voluntary standard, ASTM D-4236, and makes it mandatory for arts and crafts materials. As a result, any art material, including glazes, paints, even crayons and chalk, must carry a warning if it contains any of a number of hazardous materials, including lead. A typical lead warning will read:

> WARNING: HARMFUL IF SWALLOWED.
> MAY PRODUCE BIRTH DEFECTS.
> Contains lead.
>
> When using, do not eat, drink, or smoke.
> Wash hands immediately after use.
> Should not be used by pregnant women.
> Keep out of reach of children.
>
> Conforms to ASTM D-4236.

Note that if the phrase "Conforms to ASTM D-4236" appears by itself with no warning on the label, this means that the material has been tested and contains no harmful ingredients, including lead.

You may see the term *nontoxic* on the label. It's virtually meaningless. Prior to passage of the 1990 law mandating the ASTM standards, manufacturers were required to test for acute toxicity. A single high dose of the material was fed to animals. If more than half the animals (i.e., three out of five) died within two weeks, the product had to be labeled "toxic." If less than half (i.e., only two out of five) died within two weeks, the product could be labeled "nontoxic." In addition, CSA found that many products, especially foreign ones, carried the word *nontoxic* without the product having been tested at all.

Teachers, day-care providers, and parents all need to be aware of the many art materials that contain lead, including oil paints, crayons and chalk, spray cans of auto paint, copper enamel, and ceramic glazes. They should also know that several processes discussed earlier in the chapter, including soldering stained glass, casting lead objects, and firing lead-bearing ceramic glazes and copper enamels, release dangerous lead fumes. Papier-mâché projects should not include colored newsprint; the inks may contain lead, and instant papier-mâché mixes should be avoided, for they have been found to contain lead pigments.

An important source of safety information for all artists, hobbyists, and teachers is the Material Safety Data Sheet, which is available from manufacturers. This sheet identifies any hazardous substances that may be present in a given product, and discusses precautions and procedures for safe usage.

People involved in the theater, whether amateur or professional, need to ensure that paints and other supplies used for set and scenery fabrication are lead-free. This is especially true for stage presentations produced with or for small children.

HOW TO DISPOSE OF MATERIALS CONTAINING LEAD

Since lead is toxic, materials containing lead are hazardous; when it comes time to throw them out, they are considered hazardous waste. The EPA regulates the disposal of hazardous waste. For the most part, artists and hobbyists are exempted from the formal (and expensive) hazardous waste regulations, not because the lead products and by-products they discard are in any way safe, but because governmental management and enforcement of the disposal of consumer household waste simply isn't feasible.

That puts total responsibility on you and your conscience to dispose of lead-containing materials in as safe a manner as possible. Ask if your town or city has a collection program for household hazardous waste. This is by far the best way to dispose of solder scraps, glaze chemicals, glazes, glazed pottery, lead paints and pigments, and solvent residue from working with lead pigments. If there's no special collection set up, be sure to package your waste securely so contaminated material won't spill or blow in the wind while it's waiting to be picked up. Never burn or incinerate materials containing lead. Be sure to store these hazardous waste materials securely out of the reach of children until you can dispose of them, and don't ever pour them down the drain, either into a sewer or into a septic system.

Of course, if you avoid using materials containing lead in the first place, you eliminate the problem of disposal of hazardous waste. You, your child, and the environment will all be better off.

10

TROJAN HORSES

A child lives in a lead world.

—*J. C. Ruddock,*
"Lead Poisoning in Children," 1924

I WAS WALKING PAST a specialty shop on New York's Upper East Side one day when a miniature army in the store window caught my eye. The tiny soldiers were re-creating a scene out of Homer, busily hauling the Trojan horse to the gates of Troy. Some paint had chipped from the horse's feet, revealing a dull gray metal. And then it struck me: This little toy was in every way as treacherous as the hollow horse Agamemnon used to sneak into the House of Hector. The little horse, once a toy, now a collector's item, was cast of pure lead.

Lead enters our homes every day secreted in modern-day Trojan horses; we unwittingly carry it in, hidden away in beautiful things, in practical things, in fun things. In things ranging from fine china to the Sunday funnies; on antiques, coffee mugs, bottles of vintage wine, and even, ironically, in health and nutrition products.

It's not necessary, or even possible, to rid your home of all these things. But they do demand your awareness and need to be used with cautionary care.

ANTIQUES

Before Matthew was born, while we were outfitting the baby's room, we came across a beautiful brass and iron crib in a local antique shop.

Oh, how we wanted to buy that crib, so perfect for our turn-of-the-century home. But the price was too high, and then one day it was gone.

Just as well, I realize now, for the white paint on the iron rails almost certainly contained high levels of lead. Medical literature of the period when that crib was made is filled with horror stories of babies and children poisoned by chewing lead paint. In fact, the first childhood death recorded in our medical literature was caused by lead paint on a crib. It was described in a 1914 article in the *American Journal of Diseases of Children;* two doctors at Johns Hopkins Hospital in Baltimore wrote of a five-year-old boy who was admitted comatose with convulsions. The child was initially treated for meningitis, recovered in the hospital, and was sent home. Five months later, he was back, with the same symptoms. This time, the doctors noticed a "lead line" on the child's teeth, a telltale discoloration that pointed to lead poisoning. Blood tests confirmed the diagnosis, but the doctors wrote they were puzzled as to the source of the lead, until "he was found with his mouth covered with white lead paint which he had bitten from the railings of his crib." The little boy died a few weeks later, the first of thousands of chronicled deaths of American children from lead paint poisoning.

It's important to remember that the threat from paint is not limited to windowsills and walls; painted furniture, especially baby room furniture, poses an equal threat. Varnished furniture and accessories can also be dangerous. Varnishes often contained lead acetate, once known as "sugar of lead," to help the varnish dry. Though antique varnishes don't carry the heavy lead load of the old paints, they are another source of lead and should be kept away from kids who gnaw.

We have to recognize that antiques carry with them the burdens of past ignorance. I'm not ready to admit that the things I played and grew up with are antiques, yet many of them were coated with lead paint or printed with lead-dye inks, and some, like the toy soldiers in the shop window, were made of pure lead. Certain antiques and collectibles have no place in a home with children or where children may even visit. As far as old toys go, collect them if you must, but remember they're now for display, not play. Keep them up high, out of children's reach, and be firm when little ones beg to play with them. Keep babies and toddlers away from anything old enough to be coated with lead paint or varnish, especially if they are in the normal chewing stage or exhibit pica (see chapter 3).

CANDLES

Certain manufacturers use lead wire in the wicks of votive candles. The CPSC says two companies—Queens Braidworks, Incorporated, and the American Wick Company—use the lead wire. The lead is vaporized as the candle burns. You can identify lead-wire wicks by peeling back some of the wick's cotton braid to look for the fine wire.

CHRISTMAS ITEMS

When I was a boy, my mom and I would hang tinsel ever so carefully, one crinkled glittering strand at a time, on the tree on Christmas Eve. The tinsel weighted the branch tips down and looked for all the world like indoor icicles. I'll bet if you looked, you could still find antique tinsel in one of those stores that specialize in Christmas collectibles. Don't. This tinsel was made of strips of pure lead foil and was especially deadly for pets.

Many Christmas seasons later, a gift from Matthew's favorite playmate, a little girl up the street, drew squeals of delight when he tore off the wrapping. He's infatuated with trains, and the brightly colored box pictured an International Christmas wooden train set. As Matthew settled down to transport little sheep in the wooden cattle cars, I looked more closely at the box. A sticker had been added to the end flap, proclaiming, "No. 11113174. 21 Piece Wooden Train Set. Painted. This Is Not A Toy." There was another small-print warning on the bottom of the box, "For decorative purposes only. This is not a toy." Tell that to Matthew.

I then realized that our tree was decorated with little painted boats, toy soldiers, rocking horses, and a cornucopia of ornaments that could be mistaken for or used as toys. And I remembered how happy I was one year to find a little red metal baby carriage in Macy's Trim-a-Tree section, just the right size for a friend's daughter's dollhouse. I wondered if the paint on all these ornaments was lead-free.

I called International Silver Company in Boston, importers of the International Christmas. Customer service assured me there is no lead in the paint. I have to take their word. The un-toy is made in China, and since the package states it is not a toy, neither it nor any of the other ornament/toys have to meet the CPSC regulations limiting lead in paint.

There are two levels of potential danger associated with these toys that aren't toys. If a child in the chewing-on-everything stage gets hold of an ornament with lead paint, the level of lead ingested could be significant over even a short period of time. These children should not be allowed any access to painted ornaments.

Kids who, like Matthew, are beyond the chewing stage will still pick up a certain amount of lead as paint rubs off on their hands and is ingested through normal hand-to-mouth activity. We resolved our situation by explaining the set was a special Christmas train designed to bring the little animals to see the Christmas tree. We felt the few days of playing with it represented a low risk, and when we took the tree down, the train was packed away with the rest of the ornaments.

COSMETICS AND HAIR DYES

Cosmetic products made in foreign countries sometimes contain lead. Eye shadows made in India, known as Surma (also Ceruse or Kohl) have high levels of lead. Black Surma ranges from 12 to 32 percent lead; gray can run as high as 80 percent. If a woman uses her finger to apply eye shadow and licks her finger, she'll end up ingesting heavy doses. The lead is also absorbed through the conjunctiva, the pink part of the eyelid, although lead is not normally absorbed through the skin. Sale of these products is prohibited in the United States by the FDA, but they still show up, often mailed in by friends or relatives. If you travel, or shop in ethnic stores or markets, or a friend or relative sends you products from abroad, avoid cosmetics that may contain lead.

The FDA regulates all cosmetics sold in the United States and requires manufacturers to list ingredients on their labels. If you're a label reader, you may notice that some hair dyes contain lead acetate. The FDA says this use was approved some twelve years ago and doesn't pose a threat to the adult user. Like all such products, these dyes should be kept safely out of the reach of small children.

ETHNIC, HOME, OR FOLK REMEDIES

As managing director of the Childhood Lead Poisoning Program in Wilkes Barre, Pennsylvania, Bill Behm is used to worried calls regarding children. Still, the call from a local elementary school nurse held a surprise. She wanted him to test a powder that a fourth-grade child had been found rubbing in her eyes. The nurse said the little girl's eyes were red and inflamed; the powder came from an envelope marked "Red Lead."

Behm took a portable X-ray fluorescence machine to the school and tested the powder. It was pure lead. The little girl's parents, who are from India, were contacted, and they readily admitted to prescribing the red lead powder, actually lead tetroxide, to be used in her eyes. The girl had conjunctivitis—pinkeye—and the family believed that red lead would cure it.

When it comes to lead, ignorance is not bliss; it is deadly. Never more so than with ethnic remedies. It is heart-wrenching to know that mothers, even today, are spooning gobs of lead into children's mouths all the while thinking they are helping their sick child. It happens in Mexico and the American Southwest, and it happens in immigrant communities and homes all across the country.

Given the realities of day care, it's entirely possible that a new immigrant could end up caring for your child, either in your home or hers. You need to be aware of these lead-deadly home remedies to protect both your child and your care-provider's children. Remember: *Lead is never beneficial; it is always toxic.*

The home remedies containing lead found most frequently in the United States are *greta* (lead oxide, a yellow to grayish yellow powder) and *azarcon* (lead tetroxide, a bright reddish orange powder). *Azarcon* is known by several other names, including *alcaron, coral, liga, Maria Luisa,* and *rueda.* A third substance, *albayalde* (lead carbonate, a white powder), is also reportedly used but not as commonly. Both greta and azarcon enter the United States with Mexican immigrants. Greta seems to be preferred in Texas, azarcon in Arizona, but both have shown up throughout the Southwest. The two lead compounds are readily available in Mexico, where they are used to treat *empacho,* a blanket folk term covering vomiting and diarrhea. Greta, whose lead content has been tested between 94.1 and 97.3 percent, is sold in local hardware and supply stores in areas where it is used as a pottery glaze. Azarcon, which tests show contains 93.3 to 95 percent lead, is also distributed for industrial use, but more significantly, it's available from local drugstores and drug wholesalers. Mexican druggists use azarcon to prepare a substance called *agua de vegato,* used externally for skin problems.

The dosage given to children is staggering. The common treatment calls for anything from a pinch, "the amount you can pick up with three fingers," to as much as three teaspoons to be administered from one to five times. The use of these two deadly compounds continues in part because health professionals in Mexico don't take empacho seriously. Women report being turned away from hospitals if they say their children have empacho, despite the fact that American doctors who have examined empacho children have found legitimate concerns, usually diagnosing enteritis or gastroenteritis.

The use of lead compounds as medicine is by no means limited to Mexico; they just happen to be the remedies most commonly encountered in the United States. No one is certain how many cultures ascribe medicinal properties to the various lead compounds, but it's clear that many of them have found their way into the United States. One of the newest entries, *pay-loo-ah,* came in with the Laotian Hmong people after the Vietnam War, and there have been documented cases of pay-loo-ah lead poisoning in California and St. Paul, Minnesota. The red and orange powders are given to infants and children to combat high fevers. Lead content ranges as high as 90 percent, and officials in Minnesota found the powders readily available in local Asian food stores.

California health officials report 40 cases of elevated lead levels in one year, all attributable to lead-based ethnic remedies. In Florida, a nine-month-old Indian/Asian boy died of acute lead poisoning, the result of regular doses of lead-bearing folk remedies given as a tonic. The accompanying table lists a variety of remedies known to have high lead content, with their country or area of origin, and the malady they're most commonly used to treat.

ETHNIC REMEDIES KNOWN TO CONTAIN LEAD

NAME OF SUBSTANCE	REGION OF ORIGIN	MAX. % LEAD	MEDICINAL USE
Albayalde (a white powder)	Mexico	93%	Empacho (vomiting, colic, diarrhea, enteritis, gastroenteritis, also apathy and lethargy).
Alcaron (see Azarcon)			
Alkohl	Middle East	85%	Topical medicinal preparations; applied to umbilical stump of newborns.

NAME OF SUBSTANCE	REGION OF ORIGIN	MAX. % LEAD	MEDICINAL USE
Al Murrah	Saudi Arabia		Abdominal colic or diarrhea, stomachaches, intestinal worms.
Azarcon (red to orange powder)	Mexico	95%	Empacho
Azogue*	Mexico	—	Empacho
Bali goli (a round, flat, black bean)	Asia/India	?	Stomachache
Bint al dahab	Oman	98%	Diarrhea, constipation, abdominal colic, and general neonatal use.
Cebagn	Middle East		
Ceruse (see Surma)			
Chuifong tokuwan	Asia		
Coral (see Azarcon)			
Ghasard (a brown powder)	India	2%	Given as a tonic.
Greta (a yellow powder)	Mexico	97%	Empacho
Herbal medicines†	China	—	
Liga (see Azarcon)			
Kandu (a red powder)	Asia/India	?	Stomachache
Kohl (see Surma, Alkohl)			

NAME OF SUBSTANCE	REGION OF ORIGIN	MAX. % LEAD	MEDICINAL USE
Kushta	India/Pakistan	73%	Variety of diseases of the heart, brain, liver, and stomach. Also used as an aphrodisiac and general tonic.
Maria Luisa (see Azarcon)			
Pay-loo-ah (a red or orange powder)	Laos (Hmong)	90%	High fever, rash.
Rueda (see Azarcon)			
Saoott (see Surma)			
Surma	Asia	80%	Eye injuries. Also used as a cosmetic.
Unknown (ayurvedic substance)	Tibet	3%	Slow development.

*Azogue does not contain lead, but it is equally deadly and used to treat the same empacho symptoms. It is actually quicksilver, or liquid mercury.

†A number of Chinese herbal medicines have been found to contain lead. One brand, Poying Tan, contained 7.5 mg per dose.

Use of these ethnic remedies creates multiple problems for health providers. Low-level lead poisoning is virtually impossible to diagnose. If the child seems lethargic, the parents' natural reaction is to *increase* the dosage. As acute lead poisoning becomes less common in the United States, Western doctors have less experience with it. More time is likely to elapse before lead poisoning is diagnosed. This is another strong argument for screening, testing the blood-lead level in young children. In the meantime, it is best to check with a Western doctor before either you or your child ingest any ethnic or folk remedy. (See also "Calcium Supplements" in chapter 7 and the discussion of cosmetics in the preceding section.)

FIREPLACES AND WOODSTOVES

I lived in the rural suburbs before moving to Brooklyn. We had a wood-stove in the living room, a welcome source of warmth both figurative and literal. The stove burned all winter, and its voracious appetite kept us always on the lookout for wood. So when it came time to tear down an old garage, we saved the lumber and cut it into stove-size chunks. The old clapboard siding was especially valuable as kindling, to get the stove cranking in the morning.

Every cold morning for several years after the demise of the garage, I unwittingly turned our living room stove into a hazardous waste incinerator. The pieces of siding were loaded with a half century's worth of lead paint. Burning the paint-laden wood generated lead fumes, one of the most potent sources of lead available to the human system. Since heat doesn't break down lead (lead is an element), the lead that didn't vaporize was left in the ash, and anyone with a woodstove or fireplace knows how much ash escapes to dust the house. The ash that didn't fly around the house was dutifully carried out every Saturday morning to unintentionally pollute the backyard and garden.

In 1984, St. Louis health officials investigating a case of childhood lead poisoning found exposure to the fumes and ashes from burning lead-painted wood in a stove to be the sole cause. When the rest of the large family was tested for lead, both parents and five other children were all found to have high blood-lead levels. Curious about how common this problem might be, the St. Louis Lead Program surveyed low-income sections of the city and found that almost 10 percent of the houses heated with wood. Well over half of them contained lead-bearing woodstove ash, and analysis showed that the wood being burned contained lead concentrations as high as 30,000 ppm.

Don't burn any painted wood in a fireplace or woodstove. Treat any wood coated with what may be lead paint for what it is: toxic waste.

FISHING

Growing up, every boy I knew had a hand reel with a hook and line, a bobber, and handful of split-shot lead sinkers. The sinkers are shaped like an M&M with a groove; you put your line in the groove and then bite the sinker to squeeze it in place on the line. The soft lead was fun to bite; you could see your teeth marks in it, and it tasted kind of sweet. I know I swallowed one or two, when instead of crimping, the little sinkers shot like a watermelon seed from between my teeth.

Lead sinkers are still with us. Depending on who's providing the figures, the amount of lead used in the United States to make sinkers ranges from two to five million pounds a year. That's about to change. The EPA has banned the manufacture and sale of all lead fishing sinkers that are up to one inch in size. The ban is being phased in, to give companies time to retool, and to sell existing inventory. It's not illegal to use lead sinkers, so you don't have to throw out your existing supply.

Ironically, this is not because of their danger to children, but rather because they are deadly for certain waterfowl. EPA action came after the Environmental Defense Fund filed a petition under the Toxic Substance Control Act. The environmentalists presented evidence that trumpeter swans and common loons were being fatally poisoned by eating fishing sinkers lost in shallow waters. Other studies indicate that the sandhill crane—an endangered species—and other waterfowl from ducks and egrets to osprey and eagles are all being poisoned by eating lead sinkers.

Manufacturers anticipated the ban, and it will have little effect on most fishermen. Lead sinkers have been banned in Britain since 1987, and there are a number of viable nontoxic alternatives. Dinsmores tin sinkers, imported from Britain, have been available since the mid-1980s, and in 1993, American Sports International introduced a line of bismuth sinkers, sold through the Wal-Mart chain. Other sinkers are being made with iron and tungsten encapsulated in plastic resins and even recycled glass. An executive at one company says a major advantage to lead-free sinkers will be the safety of his employees. Workers in the mold shop currently have to undergo regular blood-lead tests. They will be safer, and since lead is often carried home in clothing, so will their families.

Lead costs 32¢ a pound; tin costs $3. Dinsmores has beaten the cost difference by designing a new dispenser for its sinkers. A 1986 survey in England found that fumble-fingered fishermen spilled four to six split-shot for every one they used! Dinsmore's new plastic container gives you one split-shot at a time, bringing the cost per use back on a par with lead.

It's also illegal to cast your own lead sinkers at home. The EPA estimates that one million fishermen make their own sinkers at home. While the ban on home casting is to keep the lead out of the environment, it will also lessen the danger of lead poisoning. Home casting exposes fishermen and their children to dangerous airborne lead particles and vapors.

FURNITURE REFINISHING

Everything we discussed about stripping finishes and paints under home renovation (see chapter 4) applies to refinishing furniture. The removal part of refinishing should be done outdoors, in the basement, or in an area that can be isolated from infants and toddlers.

Don't burn the finish off, and don't sand it off. All removal should be done over drop cloths, which should be disposed of safely once the job's complete. Wash your hands anytime you leave the project, and watch that your clothes and shoes don't carry paint residue out of the work area. Chemical paint removers, which soften and lift the paint, minimize the release of lead. Refinishers such as Formby's, which dissolve clear coatings, should not create a lead hazard.

Note: Read all labels carefully. Chemicals used in stripping and refinishing may pose other hazards not related to lead poisoning.

GUNS AND BULLETS

Bullets are made of lead. When they are fired from a gun, they release lead vapor. In a confined area, such as an indoor shooting gallery, this airborne lead level can get quite high if a lot of people are shooting and there is poor ventilation. While this is obviously not the place for little children, adults would do well to limit their exposure. It is a recognized problem for law enforcement officers, and policewomen who are planning to get pregnant or are in the early stages of pregnancy should take note.

Gallows humor refers to being shot as the ultimate form of lead poisoning. Jokes aside, bullets and bullet fragments that may be left in the body turn up repeatedly as unexpected sources of lead poisoning. The body slowly dissolves and absorbs the lead.

Some sportsmen make their own bullets, melting and casting lead and loading their own shells. Any hobby that involves molten lead poses a threat both to children and to the hobbyist (see discussion in chapter 9).

Outdoor firing ranges pump enormous quantities of lead into the environment. While it's hard to conceive of little children playing on a shooting range, it became an issue in a suburban New York county, and you need to be aware if you target-practice on your own property. Those spent bullets end up someplace, and the soft shiny globs of metal are attractive to little children. Skeet clubs typically shoot over the water, and although this practice is under attack by environmentalists because the lead shot takes an enormous toll on waterfowl, it generally doesn't pose a threat to small children, since the spent shot is usually underwater.

HAND-ME-DOWNS

Useful hand-me-downs are great whether they're family heirlooms or something resurrected from the attic. Babies are expensive, and anything new parents don't have to buy is a help. Grandma and Grandpa get a warm fuzzy feeling knowing the old bassinet will once again cradle new life. But be wary: The paint on anything more than 25 years old has to be suspect, and the older the item is, the more it should be suspected. A crib or playpen or carriage that brings lead paint into your nursery is no bargain. And if your baby is going to spend a lot of nights sleeping in the old crib at the grandparents', test the paint for lead. (See "Antiques.")

Test for lead anything painted before 1978, or else keep your young child away from it. Repainting an old crib or anything else destined for the child's room is *NOT* a solution. Little children chew, and they'll chew right through the new coat of paint. The only solution, and I almost hesitate to suggest it, is to remove the old finish and then repaint. *Before you consider this option, read chapter 4 carefully.* The dust and residue released by the removal of leaded paint is one of the worst sources of lead poisoning.

MOONSHINE

Don't laugh. My first job as a journalist was at a small North Carolina radio station. I remember being urgently pressed into duty spinning country-western tunes one Saturday morning when our disk jockey didn't show up. Turned out he'd been busted transporting cases of hootch disguised as cans of Luck's Beans!

White lightning often contains more than alcohol. The stills in the

Appalachian Hills are often built around an automobile radiator as condenser. Radiators are loaded with lead solder, which readily leaches out when exposed to alcohol-laden steam. The National Academy of Sciences analyzed 791 samples of moonshine and found traces of lead in more than 50 percent and worrisome lead levels in more than a quarter of the samples. A 1984 study of patients admitted to an Alabama hospital for chronic or acute alcoholism identified a number who gave a history of moonshine consumption. Of those tested, more than half also suffered from lead poisoning.

POOL CUE CHALK

My brother-in-law has a pool table, and it's usually a race between us and the kids to see who plays first! Matthew and his cousin delight in hitting the balls and trying to roll them into pockets. The appeal is apparently universal, an early form, my wife says, of male bonding. In Massachusetts, five-year-old David Lewis* not only liked playing with the balls; he liked the cue-tip chalk. He found the little blue cubes tasted slightly sweet (he may have been a pica child—see chapter 3) and regularly chewed on them.

David was given a routine blood-lead test when he turned six (an argument for late testing), and his lead level came back quite high. He had no history of lead poisoning, and an investigation of his home found no lead paint or other obvious source. Then his mother mentioned his peculiar penchant for pool cue chalk. Health officials tested the chalk, and it went off the scale; its lead content was in the thousands of parts per billion, more than enough to cause David's lead poisoning.

This, to me, is the scary part of lead poisoning. Sure, now we know to be careful with pool cue chalk. And everyone can be warned of the dangers of lead paint and lead dust and lead-laden soil. But what else is out there? Or in here? Seemingly innocent things like pool cue chalk carry a hidden load of deadly lead. It seems we have to discover them one-by-one, the hard way, by some child being poisoned.

SAILING

Sailboats need keels to keep from blowing over. Since lead has the highest density of all metals in common use and doesn't rust the way

*In order to protect individual's privacy, real name has been changed.

iron does, most sailboat keels are made of lead. This is perfectly harmless as long as you're sailing, but sooner or later, sailboat keels need to be sanded and repainted.

Sanding, as we stressed earlier (see chapter 4), can release deadly amounts of fine lead particles. That fine dust that gets all over you and everything else as you sand and fair your keel is a potent mix of biocidal bottom paint and lead powder.

Save the family bonding for some other activity; leave kids home while you work below the waterline. And don't take the poison home at the end of the day. Wear old clothes that you can change out of before you go home. Wash them separately. Better yet, buy a disposable coverall that can be tossed at the end of the day. For the same reason, keep your hair covered, or shampoo when you wash up before going home. For your own safety, be sure to wear a respirator when sanding and scraping, as well as when you're repainting.

SOLDERING

Building and repairing electronic items, as well as other home hobbies and home repairs that involve soldering, all involve lead. (See the cautions in chapter 9.)

TOYS

Toys don't have to be old to be dangerous. Despite everything we know about the danger lead poses to children, and despite all the laws that have been written, toys containing lead paints or inks still show up in the marketplace. Items recently recalled or removed from sale range from Barney backpacks to Barbie Tea Sets. All were manufactured overseas, most in the Far East. A list of recently recalled toys is included in appendix I.

Toy safety is largely in the hands of the CPSC, while items like tea sets, which might come into contact with food, are governed by the FDA. The 1978 law that prohibited lead in most paints includes a provision banning "toys and other articles intended for use by children that bear 'lead-containing paint'." The law goes on, in good federal fashion, for pages, carefully defining everything from children to toys. A separate law, the Hazardous Substances Act, covers crayons, chalk, and other products designed for kids. Bottom line: Anything meant for child's play cannot contain more than a trace (0.06 percent) amount of lead. (If you're repainting an old toy or a toy you've made yourself, be sure the paint you're using is lead-free. Check the label; lead content should be less than 0.06 percent. Never use marine or industrial paint on toys, cribs, or anything else a child can get his teeth or hands on.)

The CPSC depends largely on others to bring lead-bearing toys to its attention. It receives information from a Consumer Complaint Hotline; more comes from a hospital emergency room notification network; some comes from death certificates. In addition, the commission works with industry in an attempt to prevent the problem. Seminars are given annually at the February Toy Fair; other workshops are held around the country, and a *Regulated Products Handbook* is widely distributed. Manufacturers, importers, distributors, and retailers are all required to notify the CPSC within 24 hours of learning of violations of CPSC regulations, including lead in paint on a toy. Companies that have knowingly sold unsafe children's products can be hit with fines in addition to having to recall or repair the merchandise.

Most policing of the lead-in-paint toy laws is done by U.S. Customs. Customs has testing laboratories in seven port cities as well as Washington, D.C. In the New York lab, on the eighth floor of the World Trade Center, Senior Chemist Ed Sprenz demonstrates an X-ray fluorescence emissions spectrograph, a large instrument whose inside looks like a 16-cup egg poacher. The cups hold samples—of paint

---

CPSC TOY SAFETY HOTLINE

In continental U.S. .... (800) 639-CPSC

For Hearing Impaired

In Maryland .... (800) 492-8104
In rest of U.S., incl. Alaska and Hawaii .... (800) 638-8270

Or Write

Consumer Product Safety Commission
Washington, DC 20207

scrapings, or crayon, or chalk—which are x-rayed and compared with a standardized sample. A computer readout tells Sprenz whether the samples being tested contain lead.

Random and not-so-random tests are conducted on toys, chalk, crayons, finger paints, and children's books. Customs officials are obviously reluctant to discuss all the ways they intercept dangerous toys, but they say they "thrive on tips." Customs also checks import documents against records of past violations. Certain manufacturers and points of origin get close scrutiny. Art supplies being shipped from mainland China were being tested by the Los Angeles lab early in 1993 when the presence of lead was discovered. Contaminated items included colored chalk and crayons of certain colors. Boxes said the materials were "for children's use" and "for home, office, and school," and were clearly marked "nontoxic." Some 40 percent of the art supplies were contaminated with lead, making them a banned hazardous substance.

The CPSC and Customs mounted an eight-month joint investigation dubbed "Dead Lead" to halt the illegal shipments. The volume of material coming in picked up as the Christmas season approached, and before the investigation was complete, Customs had seized 18 shipments of the lead-laced crayons and chalk. Fifteen shipments were seized in Los Angeles, two in Baltimore, and one in Tampa, with the seizures totaling nearly 570,000 retail packages of children's art supplies. Several importers and a number of different factories were involved. Most of the hazardous coloring supplies were "re-exported," sent back to China to be sold somewhere else. Some were voluntarily destroyed. Customs Commissioner George Weise, father of two, called the whole thing "onerous." He was being nice.

Despite the seizure and the publicity given to it, the flood of illegal and dangerous crayons and chalk continues. Not three months after operation "Dead Lead," Arizona health officials traced a case of childhood lead poisoning to some jumbo-sized crayons the child had eaten. Arizona officials tested the crayons and found they contained 800 ppm lead. The Arizona discovery triggered a new CPSC investigation. More than 400 cases of the oversized crayons—six inches long by half an inch thick—had been imported and sold throughout the country. The jumbo crayons, made in China, were marked "nontoxic," but CPSC tests showed lead levels in red and yellow crayons ranging from 690 to 1240 ppm. The test results triggered a national alert, telling retailers to take the product off their shelves and warning parents to throw the crayons out.

The CPSC then expanded its investigation and found lead in a total of 14 different brands of Chinese-manufactured crayons. Three of the brands, imported by Concord Enterprises, Toys "R" Us, and Glory Stationery Manufacturing Company, contained enough lead to cause childhood lead poisoning all by themselves, and all of them would add unnecessarily to a child's lead intake. Eleven of the brands were ordered off the market in April 1994, and consumers were told to either return the crayons to the store or throw them out. (The CPSC has tested Crayola-brand crayons, made in the United States, and has found them to be completely lead-free.)

Getting the product off store shelves is straightforward. Getting it back from consumers is the hard part. Since there are no records of who bought the toys, the CPSC and the company involved have to rely on store signs and news releases to get the word out. Regulations specify the size and placement of store signs. The signs must make it clear what is being recalled and why, and how consumers are to be reimbursed. The CPSC usually requires the signs to remain posted for 120 days.

News releases are issued by the CPSC Office of Information and Public Affairs, which seeks to generate as much publicity about the recall as possible. (Ironically, though, it took a Freedom of Information Act request to get the CPSC list of recalled toys, which is included in appendix I.) News releases typically identify the toy, the manufacturer, the major stores selling it, and why it is being recalled. Consumers are given model and any specific identification numbers and are told how to return the toy for reimbursement.

In an effort to build toy industry cooperation, the CPSC *Handbook* stresses that consumers "no longer view product recalls in a negative light" and goes on to say that successful product recalls have often resulted in renewed consumer support and demand for the firm's products. The problem is, no one knows how successful product recalls really are. In April 1993, well into Barney-mania, the CPSC announced the recall of some 650,000 backpacks, "fanny" packs, tote bags, shoulder bags, and small handbags, most bearing the likeness of Barney and sidekick Baby Bop. (Barney, in case you're from another planet, is an overstuffed purple dinosaur that has overrun America through the medium of public television.) The Barney bags were sold all across the country is such stores as Macy's, Bloomingdales, Toys "R" Us, Kay-Bee Toys, and Sears. They were recalled because the Barney insignia and other parts of the bags contained excess levels of lead.

Was the recall successful? The CPSC doesn't know, and the distributor, Jaclyn, Inc. of West New York, New Jersey, won't tell. I called Jaclyn, to ask how the company had discovered the presence of the lead, how the problem had occurred, and how many of the recalled items were actually recovered. Two weeks and several phone calls later, I got stonewalled. "There is no one at Jaclyn," I was informed, "who can answer your questions."

What can a parent do? Buying name-brand merchandise at major stores is no guarantee; witness the recalls of merchandise carrying the Barney, Barbie, Cabbage Patch Kids, and Holly Hobbie names. Without meaning to be protectionist, I suggest you look for a "Made in America" label; domestic manufacturers are less likely to break federal law. Make a point to check the bulletin boards at the entrance to your local toy store. Ask the store manager if there have been any recent toy recalls, and not only for lead. Read the parenting magazines such as *Child* and *Working Mother* which regularly carry notices about toy recall.

When it comes to crayons and chalk, the CPSC tells parents (and schoolteachers, day-care providers, etc.) to look for a label saying: "Conforms to ASTM D-4236." ASTM is the American Society for Testing and Materials; it sets standards for safety, and D-4236 is its standard for safety in crayons and chalk. It is supposed to guarantee that the product is safe, but when the CPSC investigated Chinese crayon imports during 1994, one of the brands containing the highest amount of lead also carried the ASTM label on its package along with the word *nontoxic*. Clearly, if a company is willing to violate federal safety laws and risk the health of children, it's not likely to hesitate at a little false labeling. Not one of the companies involved was fined or subjected to legal action. The CPSC explains that it's reluctant to prosecute first-time offenders and companies that cooperate in a recall action.

It's time for the federal government to get tough with companies that import and sell these products. Given the Chinese manufacturers' blatant scorn for our laws and our safety, parents should boycott any coloring supplies imported from China. The crayon problem in April 1994 was no isolated accident; it involved 11 brands and 700 million crayons, and it followed years of similar incidents. Almost all of the millions of lead-tainted crayons were, by the admission of the sellers, off the shelves and in our homes by the time the CPSC warning was issued. The government told us to either return them or throw them out. That's good advice, but how many of the crayons are still in a returnable, identifiable box? And how many people are going to schlep back to a store to return a $2 box of crayons? My guess is that very few of those 700 million will be returned. You and I take the hit; the stores and importers keep the profits. Until the CPSC hits them with fines—fines big enough to hurt—these companies will continue to put our children unnecessarily at risk. Importing and selling crayons contaminated with lead is no paperwork violation; there is an infant in Phoenix, Arizona, who is lead poisoned because these crayons were brought into the United States.

TRAVEL

Not all countries are as aware of the dangers of lead poisoning as we are. Toys may be painted with lead-base paint or may even be cast of pure lead. Pottery, ceramics, and china may all contain lead glazes that will leach. Canned foods and drinks may contain lead solder. Be especially leery of local cosmetics and native remedies which may contain extremely high levels of lead.

Be careful what you bring home! And if you will be taking young children abroad for an extended period, you need to conduct the same kind of survey that you did at home, paying full attention to lead paint and lead-paint dust, but also being aware of sources of lead unique to the local culture or country.

WEIGHTS

Ever make a suggestion that something "went over like a lead balloon"? As everyone knows, lead is heavy. It's the most dense of all common metals, weighing almost half again as much as an equal-sized lump of iron. In addition, it does not break down and stain in the same way as iron does when it rusts. As a result, lead is useful simply as a weight. In addition to sinkers (see "Fishing"), lead weights can be found in the bottom of everything from shower curtains to the living room draperies. Lead shot shows up in things as diverse as paperweights and the bases of tape dispensers.

These uses pose no hazard as long as the lead is encapsulated. However, if the lead shot spills, or the curtain rips and the lead weight falls out, these objects are prime candidates to end up in the mouths of infants and toddlers.

Avoid the use of lead whenever possible. Substitute steel shot for lead shot. Where lead weights are sewn into curtains and draperies, make certain they can't come free and fall out. Dispose of unneeded lead weights and shot carefully.

One final note: I was amazed to learn that those little lead soldiers that started me thinking about ways lead sneaks into the home are still being made today, and they are still available as children's toys! A CPSC Summary of Mandatory Standards, while saying that the use of metallic lead in toys for small children should be discouraged, states that medical evidence doesn't indicate the need for regulatory action. The CDC concludes: "Metallic lead or elemental lead is less hazardous than many of the lead salts used in paint prior to the ban. Since metallic lead does not have a tendency to flake or peel like paint, it is less likely to be ingested."

Tell that to a toddler who chews. How do you explain a government that will ban lead fishing sinkers but still allow children's toys to be made of lead?

11

BUYING AND SELLING; RENTING AND LEASING

Children are being used as the
barometer of lead in the environment.

—Dr. Howard Moenson
American Academy of Pediatrics

WE HAD A PROFESSIONAL ENGINEER survey our house before we bought it. His report ran for several pages—a first-floor rear windowsill needs replacement, weather-strip the rear door, the main girder is oak, and so on—but there was no mention of lead paint or the risk of lead poisoning.

Five years ago, for most of us, the dangers posed by exposure to lead were still over the horizon. Low-level lead poisoning was becoming a hot topic in the medical journals, but for people like us who were buying a home, the only problem presented by peeling paint was that it needed to be scraped, the only threat posed by the lead water-service line was the possibility it might leak. And so we, and the Roseberrys and Sheehans and countless others like us, bought our lead-laden houses and moved in to raise our children, blissfully ignorant of what lurked in the walls and pipes and garden soil. Our children would be modern-day canaries in the mine; their becoming poisoned would alert us, after the fact, to the presence of lead in our homes.

That is changing. People are becoming more aware, are starting to ask questions. Engineers are beginning to include lead tests in their inspections. Protection is starting to be written into law. We are finally moving to true prevention, to the identification of lead hazards—especially lead-based paint hazards—*before* they can poison our children. In so doing, we're creating market forces that will encourage lead-paint abatement.

HELP IS ON THE WAY WITH TITLE X

The driving piece of national legislation, known as Title X (Title Ten), puts major protections into effect in October 1995. Officially titled the Residential Lead-based Paint Reduction Act, it's going to put the residential lead-paint problem squarely on the front burner. Title X applies to *all* housing, including owner-occupied and privately owned rental property, built before 1978. It marks the first time that federal legislation has moved into the private housing arena, and it will insert the issue of lead poisoning into almost every real estate transaction in the country. From renting an apartment to buying or selling a house, a co-op, or a condominium, Title X turns "caveat emptor" on its ear. The governing principle in housing transactions is becoming "make the buyer aware." Some key provisions:

■ The buyer or renter must be given a pamphlet on the hazards of lead paint, now being developed by EPA with input from HUD and HHS.

■ The buyer or renter must be informed of any lead-based paint or any known lead-paint hazard.

■ The home buyer will have a 10-day period in which to inspect the property for lead hazards.

In addition, home buyers have to sign a statement saying they've received the required pamphlet, been given 10 days to look for lead paint, and that they've read and understood the following warning statement:

Every purchaser of any interest in residential real property on which a residential dwelling was built prior to 1978 is notified that such property may present exposure to lead from lead-based paint that may place young children at risk of developing lead poisoning. Lead poisoning in young children may produce permanent neurological damage, including learning disabilities, reduced intelligence quotient, behavioral problems, and impaired memory. Lead poisoning also poses a particular risk to pregnant women. The seller of any interest in residential real property is required to provide the buyer with any information on lead-based paint hazards from risk assessments or inspections in the seller's possession and notify the buyer of any known lead-based paint hazards. A risk assessment or inspection for possible lead-based paint hazards is recommended prior to purchase.

Violations of the notification requirements give the buyer or renter the right to sue, and liability applies not only to the seller or landlord but also to any real estate agent or management firm. The idea is to create a market force that will drive reduction of the lead-paint hazard. It's already starting to work. While Title X disclosure was still 18 months off, a front-page story in the *New York Times* Real Estate section, headlined "Lead Paint Moves Up as Housing Issue," surveyed the growing awareness of lead-paint hazards and their financial implications. By making lead paint a negative factor at the time of sale, disclosure is creating a market incentive for abatement. If lead-free housing is worth more at closing, it makes sense to spend money to remove lead.

If you're about to buy a home, there's no need to wait for Title X to kick in. By all means have it tested for lead, not only for lead-based paint but for potential lead leaching from the plumbing system. Depending on how much is involved, lead-paint abatement can make a new furnace look downright cheap. Dealing with lead plumbing can be expensive too; we were told it will cost some $5,000 to replace the service line coming into our house. These are things that affect the net value, and should therefore affect the price, of a house (or condo or co-op). If you know before you buy that there's lead paint to abate, the cost becomes negotiable; find out later, and the cost could drive you into bankruptcy.

Although disclosure is important for renters, too, potential tenants have neither the leverage nor the options of home buyers. Many renters will face take-it-or-leave-it situations, and for the majority of people who rent in urban areas, they can't leave it because there's no place else to go. The pool of affordable rental housing is both small and polluted; the fact of life for most low- and many moderate-income families in our older cities is that any housing they can afford will likely contain lead-based paint.

That doesn't mean you throw up your hands and do nothing. If you have to rent an apartment or home that contains lead-based paint, the awareness of the potential for lead-paint poisoning gives you the opportunity (and responsibility) to practice the many prevention techniques discussed in chapter 2. Though abatement is the only long-term remedy for lead-paint hazards, there is much the educated parent can do to lessen the level of a child's lead exposure.

You should also learn if there are any laws or regulations covering lead-based paint where you'll be living. There is no federal law requiring the abatement of lead-based paint in private housing. That responsibility is left up to the states, and the result is a patchwork of protection. Two of the states providing greater protection are Massachusetts, which for years has required professional abatement of any housing where a child is found to have an elevated lead level, and Maryland, which requires lead-paint inspection whenever a house or apartment is sold or rented. (More on Maryland later in the chapter.) At the opposite end of the scale are the majority of states that have no regulations whatsoever dealing with owner responsibility for the lead-paint hazard. The law may even vary from city to city within a state. Your best source of information should be your local public health agency. Or you may get information from the source listed for your state in appendix D.

Residents of public housing fare a little better. Title X requires that all public housing units built before 1960 be tested for lead paint. That testing has to be completed by the end of 1995, and tenants have to be notified if lead-based paint is found. There's also a schedule for testing units built between 1960 and 1978 that will have all those units tested by the end of 2001. The law also requires testing for lead before any paint-disturbing renovation work is started, and any rehabilitation work will automatically trigger the reduction or abatement of lead-paint hazards. Abatement of lead paint in government housing is discussed later in this chapter.

LANDLORD LIABILITY

While the disclosure provisions apply to rental situations, there is no requirement for a formal lead-paint hazard warning in the lease. When Title X was drafted, it was felt that including such a warning would work against the rights of the tenant. Much as cigarette companies now invoke required cigarette label warnings to defend themselves in health-related lawsuits, landlords sued over the lead poisoning of a child might hide behind the warning, claiming parents knew the risk and accepted it. (*Under no circumstances should you sign a lease in which you acknowledge or in any way take responsibility for the presence of lead-based paint.* Should your child become lead poisoned, you will have signed away all rights to recover damages.)

Landlord liability has become an important factor in the rental market. Thousands of lawsuits have been filed in cities across the nation. Most of these claim landlord negligence: for failure to test for the presence of lead-based paint, failure to warn of the presence of lead-based paint, failure to maintain property, failure to abate lead-based paint or even worse, failure to properly abate lead-based paint, and/or failure to comply with whatever lead-paint statutes, regulations, ordinances, or codes might be in effect.

Courts are typically finding landlords liable if (1) the child ingested lead from paint in the landlord's building, (2) the child was injured by the lead, and (3) the landlord was negligent. Negligence means the landlord knew, or should have known, that there was a lead-paint hazard in the building and didn't do anything about it. With the attention given to lead poisoning and lead-based paint in recent years, it's become difficult for a landlord to claim ignorance of the hazard.

For families of lead-poisoned children, a lawsuit offers the hope of recovering the cost of medical treatment and special education, if it's needed, as well as damages for the loss of what might have been. For activists, lawsuits are a tool for change. John McConnell, Jr., an attorney in a series of lawsuits targeting 28 landlords, calls the suits "a shot across the bow in the war against lead poisoning. The tort system," he says, "is powerful in bringing about change."

The shots can be big ones. A Milwaukee court has ordered the American Family Insurance Company to make monthly payments to a five-year-old boy for the rest of his life. The little boy was found to be lead poisoned, and the city ordered the owners of the apartment where he lived to abate the lead paint. They did, by scraping. The child's lead level shot from the low 30s µg/dl to the 80s µg/dl. He has been diagnosed with attention deficit disorder with hyperactivity and has suffered permanent neurological damage. The settlement could cost the insurance company $1.5 million.

In a New York City case, important for its many ramifications, the family of a lead-poisoned child was awarded $1.7 million. The family claimed their dwelling had peeling lead-based paint and that, despite numerous complaints, the landlord did nothing about it. The case, *Miller v. Beaugrand,* has an impact that goes far beyond the size of the award. New York City had taken over the property in a foreclosure proceeding, and the city didn't abate the lead condition until some four months after taking title. As a result, the court held the city 20 percent liable for the child's injury and therefore 20 percent liable for the damage award. In the end, because the private landlord went bankrupt, the city had to pay the entire award amount.

The city got caught by what's called *joint and several liability*, which means in essence that anyone who can be shown to have any legal connection to an offending property (or product) can be held liable for the damage or injury it causes. Lenders who had little to fear from the risk of lead poisoning have a lot to fear from the risk of joint and several liability. One result is that banks are starting to look for lead-based paint before they write loans on residential property. This can be good when it brings about abatement, but, too often, homeowners who need financing to abate a lead-paint problem can't get it.

Settlements like the one in Milwaukee have insurance companies scrambling to write lead liability out of their policies. In New York State alone, the Department of Insurance has given permission for 21 commercial insurers to completely exclude lead liability coverage from their policies. Another 18 companies want to do the same thing. Many don't need permission; their policies already have pollution exclusion clauses, and the courts have generally interpreted these to exclude lead-based-paint claims.

The result of these factors in combination has been to thrust thousands of low-income rental units into liability limbo. Owners, afraid or unable to rent properties, stop making mortgage and tax payments and eventually abandon them. Neither the banks nor the city dare foreclose, so the property sits ownerless and vacant until time and vandals do it in.

For the special situation that arises when the property owner is the federal government, see the discussion later in this chapter.

LIABILITY OF INDUSTRY

Certainly the paint manufacturers and the lead companies have a legal connection to the offending product; they, after all, made and sold and promoted it. The problem comes in proving just whose paint is on the wall. Building owners have tried to get around this dilemma by charging collective liability and suing all the manufacturers, but courts have rejected the concept. Even when landlords can show through purchase records what company's paint was used, they run into statute-of-limitations problems. Residential use of lead-based paint was banned nationally in 1977, earlier in some cities, and building owners trying to sue find their legal clock has run out.

Clever lawyers in New York recently found a way around both problems. In *City of New York v. Lead Industries Association, Inc.*, an appeals court found that manufacturers of lead-based paint could be held jointly and severally liable, not for making the toxic product but for concealing its hazards, misleading the public and the government, and marketing unsafe products. The city got around the statute of limitations by demonstrating that it learned of the fraud only recently, during other legal proceedings.

The lead industry may have stubbed its toe in Massachusetts. Lawyers for a lead-poisoned child, unable to prove which brand of paint was involved, sought damages from the five companies that supplied virtually all the lead used in the manufacture of paint. They asked that the damages be assessed on the basis of the market share each company had at the time the paint was made. As part of their defense, the companies argued that "market-share damages" was a novel legal concept more appropriately the domain of the legislature than the courts.

Attorneys active in the field of childhood lead poisoning took the hint, drafted a bill, and went looking for someone to introduce it. They looked for a long time. Then they found Patricia Jehlen, mother of three, all of whom, she says, had elevated levels of lead in their blood back when 40 µg/dl was the official level of concern (it's now 10 µg/dl). The two-term representative introduced "market-share" legislation that would allow both the families of lead-poisoned children and landlords required to abate lead-based paint to sue the lead manufacturers. If the court decided that a plaintiff deserved damages and it couldn't be proved which company's paint was at fault, the judge would assess damages to each of the five lead manufacturers in proportion to their market share at the time the paint was made.

The leadership of both parties opposed Jehlen's bill. The cochairman of the Judiciary Committee argued on the House floor that market-share liability would "change radically the tort and product-liability law in this state," and the Judiciary Committee recommended the bill not pass. But by a vote of 87–53, the full House voted to ignore the Judiciary Committee's recommendation, and it took up Jehlen's bill.

The final vote in favor of the bill was even more lopsided, but time ran out, and the session ended without Senate action. Jehlen's bill has been refiled in both the House and Senate, but the lead industry has hired the best lobbyists Beacon Hill has to offer, starting with a former president of the Senate. The House leadership, mindful of the support the bill has on the floor, is maneuvering to keep it from coming to a vote, but Pat Jehlen remains optimistic. "These companies," she says, "knew they were selling a dangerous product all the while they were promoting lead paint."

LEAD PAINT, HOUSING, AND THE FEDERAL GOVERNMENT

The owner of the house that poisoned the two Roseberry children knew about the presence of lead paint and knew better than most the risk the paint posed to the family. The Roseberrys bought their house from the federal government.

"The government told us the property had to meet strict government codes before it could let us take possession. The septic system was old, so the government paid to hook the house to the municipal sewer. It put in a new hot-water heater, fixed the furnace, repaired broken windows, installed ground-fault outlets in the bathroom. The government even replaced a toilet bowl that had cracked while the house sat vacant. We felt," Sandra says, "like, oh, wow! We're buying from the government." The Roseberrys didn't think twice about their contract. It specified they were buying the house "as is."

They purchased the house from the Veteran's Administration—the VA had taken possession in a foreclosure action. Later, after their children became lead poisoned, after the state declared the house unsafe for human habitation, Sandra asked the VA, why? Why, when they did all the piddling repairs, did they ignore, despite clear HUD guidelines, lead paint, the greatest hazard of all? Came the answer: Those are HUD guidelines, and we're the VA.

Estimates for abating the lead-based paint exceeded the original price of the house, and the VA refused to hear of the problem. The family tried to sue in First Circuit Court, but the judge ruled they didn't meet the criteria for suing the U.S. government. By now separated—not uncommon in families torn by the emotions and pressures associated with having lead-poisoned children—and in bankruptcy, the Roseberrys tried to appeal. The judge in the First Circuit Court of Appeals wouldn't even hear the case. "As is," he said, "means 'as is'."

Sandra eventually contacted Don Ryan at the Alliance To End Childhood Lead Poisoning. Ryan called Congressman Tom Lantos of California. Lantos was chairman of a Government Operations subcommittee that happened to be looking into the effectiveness of HUD's lead-paint guidelines. Lantos called Sandra Roseberry. He asked her to testify before Congress. Her testimony, and the testimony of other families betrayed by trusting the government, led to enactment of a crucial section of Title X.

The old statute called on Uncle Sam to use common sense when it came to lead paint, requiring the government to "eliminate as far as practical immediate hazards" from any housing that it was associated with. The new law forces the federal government to be a responsible property owner, realtor, and landlord. The government will have to abate lead paint in any pre-1960 housing that the government sells or helps to finance or rehabilitate, including properties sold by the Federal Deposit Insurance Corporation and the Resolution Trust Corporation. There's one catch, though, and it's a big one: Abatement is subject to Congress making the funds available.

Title X also brings lead-paint protection to people living in military and other federal housing. Federally-owned housing becomes subject not only to the terms of Title X, but also to state and local laws, even if more stringent.

Title X also addresses the need for standards in every phase of the abatement process. Standards for licensing contractors, certifying laboratories, accrediting training programs, protecting workers, protecting residents while work is in progress, and reducing risks caused by renovation and remodeling—all are finally being codified in a HUD document tentatively titled "Guidelines for the Evaluation and Control of Lead-Based Paint Hazards in Housing" due to be issued in January 1995. It will be the mandate for federal contracting, and it's certain to become the model for the rest of the nation.

FUNDING FOR LEAD-PAINT ABATEMENT

Congress appropriated $150 million for lead-paint abatement in private housing in 1994, up from $100 million the year before and triple what was available in 1992. That may sound like a lot of money, but it amounts to about $7.50 for each of the 20 million housing units identified by HUD as having elevated lead-dust levels or where lead-based paint is visibly peeling and chipping. That's not enough to buy a quart of paint remover, and there's another 37 million houses and apartment units where the lead-based paint isn't peeling; it's just being ground into fine lead dust.

The federal money is channeled through a HUD grants program designed to reduce lead-based paint hazards in low-income, privately owned housing. The grants go to states or local governments to be used for individual grants, loans, loan guarantees, and interest write-downs or subsidies. As small as the pie is, not all of it goes to abate lead paint. Up to 10 percent can be carved off for local administrative expenses. More can be used for everything from public education to the blood-lead monitoring of abatement workers. Clearly, more money is needed.

But where, in this age of deficit fighting and budget cutting, is the money going to come from? New Jersey Senator Bill Bradley and Maryland Congressman Benjamin Cardin think it should come from a tax on the use of lead. The two legislators introduced similar bills in the Senate and House which would create a $1-billion-a-year trust fund for the abatement of lead-based paint hazards. The money would come from an excise tax of 45¢ per pound on newly produced (or imported) lead. The excise would add about $8 to the cost of a car battery not made from recycled lead. The justice of this "polluter pays" approach would seem obvious. Lead is the known toxin; its pervasiveness today is the direct result of the industry's aggressive promotion of lead in paint, despite mounting evidence of its deadly toll on children. Yes, the tax would ultimately be passed on to us as consumers. But we would be reminded that there is "a price to pay" when using a toxic substance like lead; we would be encouraged to seek alternatives to lead whenever possible, and to conserve and recycle lead when it must be used. The incentive to recycle lead would be an important side benefit of the legislation, keeping lead out of the waste stream and, ultimately, the environment.

As executive director of the Alliance To End Childhood Lead Poisoning, Don Ryan lobbies Capitol Hill on behalf of children. He finds himself locking horns with "an extraordinarily aggressive" lead industry lobby. He should not be surprised, given the lead industry's earlier success in holding off any legislation against lead paint for decades — from the 1920s to the 1970s (see discussion in chapter 3).

The lead industry mounted a campaign of dis-information to fight the proposed lead tax. Typical was a front-page *Wall Street Journal* article headlined "Dogma in Doubt." The article builds fallacious arguments on carefully selected "facts" to question both the extent of lead's risk and the need to remove lead paint. It argues against blood testing to screen children for lead poisoning by quoting a pediatrician at an upscale California clinic who hasn't "seen a child sick from lead poisoning in years." I'm sure he hasn't. Since there are no symptoms for low-level lead poisoning, if you don't test for it, you won't see it; that's the point of screening. In another bit of sophistry, the fact that improper lead-paint abatement can increase a child's risk of lead poisoning was presented as an argument against all lead-paint abatement.

While lead apologists spread "lead poisoning is a problem of the past" hyperbole, the lead lobby moved on Capitol Hill. Sophisticated to the point that many in Washington don't even know it exists, lead industry lobbyists used surrogates to spread the industry message; so every member of the critical House Ways and Means Committee got a visit from a local business leader, often with a local union leader in tow, chanting the mantra that a lead tax would drive them out of business and put whole communities out of work.

It's nonsense, of course. For the principal users of lead, there is presently no substitute. Lead-acid batteries can't be made out of tin. And when a car battery dies, it has to be replaced, right now, and it has to be replaced with another lead-acid battery. No excise tax in the world can change that. The congressional Joint Committee on Taxation, which studies the impact of proposed taxes, found that the Bradley-Cardin lead tax would "cause little economic distortion," meaning no loss of jobs. But the damage was being done.

Efforts to fund lead-based paint abatement melded naturally into the larger health-care reform movement, and Cardin's bill was absorbed into health reform legislation being considered by a House Ways and Means Health subcommittee. Don Ryan and the Alliance worked to counter the lead lobby, at one point digging deeply into its pockets to finance a full-page ad in *Roll Call*, Capitol Hill's newspaper. "Congress," the ad cried, "It's time to put children's health interests ahead of lead's special interests. It's time for the lead industry to help pay for the damage it has caused." The ad, with help from the Building and Construction Trades Department of the AFL-CIO, pointed out that funding lead abatement, which is notably labor intensive, would create an estimated 27,000 jobs.

When the health-care reform package finally emerged, the abatement trust fund was still there, but it had been cut in half, and the lead industry was off the hook. Instead of a lead tax, the representatives invoked logic indigenous only to Capitol Hill and agreed to finance the removal of lead-based paint through a four-cent-a-pack tax on cigarettes!

Don Ryan will take abatement funding wherever he can get it, but taxing cigarettes bothers him, in part because the legislation has a long way to go before passage and the illogic of the tax makes it vulnerable, but mostly because the lead industry is not held accountable. This industry, he says, "needs to be part of the solution. They need to clean up the mess they've made." The lead-paint abatement trust fund died in 1994 along with the rest of the health care bill. Both Cardin and Bradley plan to reintroduce their legislation in the next Congress. I hope that by the time you read this, Congress will have acted to provide a greater base of funding for the abatement of lead-based paint— ideally, one tied to the use of lead. But don't count on it.

THE AFFORDABLE HOUSING DILEMMA

Lead paint and childhood lead poisoning are interrelated problems everywhere, but nowhere are they as epidemic as in the poorest sections of our old cities. And nowhere are they more intractable. Abatement options and opportunities disappear when you cross the poverty line. Money is one thing common to the forces that drive lead-paint abatement. Incentives, be they positive or negative, all depend on it. Homeowners who want to protect their children and landlords who want to be law abiding both need access to money. The freedom to move requires a certain level of income. Tax credits are an incentive only if you owe taxes; most low-income homeowners do not. With no money or value at stake, fines become meaningless, and liability suits are neither enticing to attorneys nor threatening to landlords. In too many urban "lead belts," the money just is not there.

Baltimore is a typical old city. The bulk of its housing dates from before 1950 and is loaded with lead paint. Large sections of the city are impoverished. Childhood lead poisoning is rampant; 50 percent of the children test above 10 μg/dl, 40 percent above 20 μg/dl. Dr. Julian Chisholm of Baltimore's Kennedy Krieger Institute is conducting a multimillion-dollar study of the new chelating agent Succimer there in part because the city has a ready pool of young patients.

Baltimore's interest in lead poisoning goes back to the 1930s, when it established the nation's first lead poisoning prevention program, including free lab analysis for blood-lead tests. Lead paint was banned from public housing. But, as elsewhere, the city's private housing was loaded with lead paint. Because the city was one of the first to screen for lead poisoning, Baltimore became one of the first to realize the scope of the problem, and Maryland put a strong lead abatement law in place. And then, because it was so poor, Baltimore became the first to reach abatement gridlock.

The numbers tell it all. Full-scale lead abatement of a typical Balti-more row house can cost anywhere from $7,000 to $12,000. The row houses sell, if you can find a buyer, for $12,000 to $15,000. No bank will loan money on the basis of numbers like that. With most tenants earning less than $10,000 a year, rents cap out at $225 to $250 a month. There is no way to amortize abatement. Baltimore's inner city has more corporations per block than the state of Delaware; landlords, unable to get liability insurance, have incorporated each house sepa-rately. No tort lawyer is going to bring a suit that could win him a $15,000 house carrying a $9,000 mortgage requiring $10,000 of abatement. And if the city slaps a citation on the door, the owner walks away. With some 3,000 lead-paint suits pending, a survey found the number of vacant or abandoned houses in Baltimore had topped 7,000 and was climbing. For inner-city Baltimore, and large sections of many other American cities, lead paint and childhood lead poisoning is not just a major health problem; it has become a housing problem.

Like aging heavyweights at the end of a long bout, opposing forces in Baltimore finally ran out of fight. Property owners and health advo-cates, state agencies and the city government—even the paint indus-try—all agreed they were in gridlock. And that created an opportunity. The governor appointed a 15-member commission, all key players, and named the dean of the University of Maryland Law School to chair it. The challenge: to find a self-supporting no-fault compensation system and to find some way of making old housing safe without bankrupting landlords and forcing abandonment.

Maryland's Lead Paint Poisoning Commission was appointed in September 1992. By December 1993, it had drafted model legislation, and five months later the General Assembly completed action and Gov-ernor Donald Schaefer had signed it into law.

Compromise was key to the fast action. Landlords were willing to make their units safer, but they wanted to minimize costs and they needed to limit their liability. Health advocates, given the Hobson's choice of health or housing, agreed to target the greatest hazards first. Thus properties built before 1950 get first attention. Common sense came into play: Visibly dangerous conditions have to be handled im-mediately, but unless a child is found to be lead poisoned, landlords are allowed to delay more extensive abatement until the property turns over, with a break between occupants. This flexible time frame saves landlords the considerable extra expense of relocating tenants during abatement without unduly slowing the larger process. National figures show that 38 percent of all rental property turns over every year; at that rate, lead exposure in most target housing will have been reduced within five to six years. Abatement requirements are relaxed. Most intact lead paint can be left in place. Resources are spent removing or capping paint that's accessible to small children and preventing the creation of lead-paint dust. Special attention is given to floors, making them smooth and sealing them so they can be kept clean. When the work is done, the unit is thoroughly washed and HEPA vacuumed.

In return for doing all this work, landlords get liability protection. If a child in an abated home is found to have a blood-lead level over 25 μg/dl, the landlord is responsible for the cost of relocating the child into a truly lead-free environment and for a certain amount of medical expense, but he is protected from the enormous costs of legal action and the threat of a million-dollar settlement.

There is a lot more to it, of course; the law runs on for 77 pages, and there are many devils in the details, including inspection and testing. And although everyone agreed that window replacement was desirable, the dollars weren't there and the issue was set aside for later discussion. The new Maryland law is not perfect; children's advocates say it goes too far in protecting landlords. Nick Farr, director of the National Center for Lead-Safe Housing in nearby Columbia, Maryland, and a commission member, doesn't support the law for this reason but admits it's going "to make a lot more homes a lot more lead-safe."

State legislatures all across the country, driven in part by Title X requirements for contractor licensing and training, in part by public pressure and by growing liability issues, are grappling with many aspects of the lead issue. The National Conference of State Legislatures said at last count there were 223 bills relating to lead pending nationwide.

The push for legislation to control lead exposure has the benefit of a model state law to work from. The draft "Lead Poisoning Prevention Act" is a joint project of the Alliance To End Childhood Lead Poisoning, based in Washington, D.C., and the Conservation Law Foundation, located in Boston. While the model could be adopted as a stand-alone turnkey lead prevention package, its 52 different sections provide language to cover everything from screening and abatement to assessment and liability. It emphasizes cost-effective prevention and concentrates on the control and elimination of the sources of lead poisoning, primarily lead-based paint, and is a useful tool to anyone interested in legislating lead-paint protection.

Copies of the "Lead Poisoning Prevention Act" are available from the Alliance To End Childhood Lead Poisoning, and copies of the "Maryland Lead Paint Poisoning Commission Report" are available from the National Center for Lead-Safe Housing. Nominal fees may be charged. Addresses for both organizations are in appendix B.

While the disclosure component of Title X gives buyers and renters important new protections—I certainly wish we had known up-front of the existence, and danger, of lead paint in our house—the most influential element of the complex law may well be the simple booklet EPA is writing about the dangers of lead-based paint. It's a 20-page wake-up call, broadcasting the warning that lead is dangerous and that lead-based paint is a threat to your family's physical and economic health. The message is hard to ignore, and EPA estimates that 20 million of these booklets will be put in the hands of prospective renters and buyers every year. Don't underestimate the impact. Termites have yet to poison their first child, but people understand they are an economic threat. As a result, there isn't a home sold today that isn't inspected for termites; if found, they're exterminated and their damage abated.

   With 20 million people a year about to be put on notice about the many costs of lead poisoning, it shouldn't be long before lead-based paint gets at least the same attention.

ENDNOTE

THE LARGER ISSUE

*The tragedy is that of bright, healthy
children whose intellectual abilities are
permanently dimmed and scholastic
performance is forever limited.*

—*J. Julian Chisholm, M.D.*
Kennedy Krieger Institute

FOR YEARS, lead poisoning has been seen as a ghetto problem, a
malady of minorities and the poor. While we're learning now that we
all share the risk—plenty of middle- and upper-class kids live in houses
with lead-paint dust and lead-tainted water, surrounded by lead-contaminated soil—there is no escaping the fact that the children of poverty—living in dilapidated housing with peeling, flaking paint—are in
double jeopardy. As a group, they run a higher risk of being lead poisoned, and when poisoned, they run the risk of significantly higher
blood-lead levels. Connect the fact that 50 percent of inner-city children suffer lead poisoning with what we know about the effects of lead
on intelligence, behavior, and the capability to learn, and you unearth
the taproot of the seemingly intractable problems of the ghetto.

Lead in paint is not just a health issue. It is a social issue. Lead is a
key to breaking the tight cycle of poverty with which we have struggled
for decades: Poverty exposes children to lead; lead retards the child's
mental and behavioral growth; the adolescent drops out of school; the
grown child is returned to poverty, and the cycle begins anew.

"We have failed to confront the role lead plays," Bailus Walker
says. Walker is dean of the public-health school at the University of

Oklahoma, former commissioner of public health in Massachusetts, and chairman of the board of directors of the Alliance To End Childhood Lead Poisoning.

"We want to blame the one-parent family and a whole range of other factors when little Johnny raises hell in class," he says. "No one says, 'test for lead in little Johnny's blood.' " The study, which finds lead poisoning to be a consistent precursor of crime, holds little surprise for Walker: "Test a violent adolescent," he says, "and you'll find elevated levels of lead."

Children must be screened for lead. The best schools and the best teachers in all the world cannot teach and may not even be able to control a child whose brain has been damaged by lead. Early screening can detect lead poisoning in time to prevent the worst damage.

Screening brings us back to the fact that lead poisoning must be prevented. In the inner city, that means wholesale lead-paint abatement. Legislation to establish a lead-abatement trust fund, introduced by Senator Bill Bradley (D-New Jersey) and Representative Benjamin Cardin (D-Maryland), is supported by the construction industry, which anticipates the creation of thousands of inner-city jobs, and by health officials and children's advocates. However, the potentially powerful voice of the education lobby has been sadly silent, and funding for lead abatement has been vehemently and effectively opposed by the lead industry.

Those who argue against abating lead paint as public policy say we cannot afford the bill. Yet we are paying it every day. We pay for lead poisoning in everything from lost productivity to overflowing prisons, and we keep on paying generation after generation. Julian Chisholm, who has crusaded against lead paint for decades, makes the point that lead-paint abatement in the inner city is a one-time-only cost that is repaid over and over. Low-income housing units turn over quickly, so the abatement of lead paint in a single housing unit protects a succession of children who will move in and out over the years to come.

Perhaps the greatest impediment to establishment of a trust fund to abate lead paint is public indifference. Many members of congress say they find it difficult to support funding lead abatement when their constituency is quiet on the subject.

Screening children for lead poisoning could change that. When I learned that Matthew, that *my* son, was lead poisoned, I was quickly motivated to act, first to protect him, then to protect others. As millions of other parents are given similar news, they too will confront the threat posed by this silent hazard. I hope they will speak out, to demand that we face up to the legacy of lead.

APPENDIX A

ALPHABET SOUP!

ANSI	American National Standards Institute
ASTM	American Society for Testing and Materials
ATSDR	U.S. Agency for Toxic Substances and Disease Registry
CDC	U.S. Centers for Disease Control
CERCLIS	Comprehensive Environmental Response, Compensation, and Liability Information System
CPSC	U.S. Consumer Product Safety Commission
CSA	Center for Safety in the Arts
EDF	Environmental Defense Fund
EPA	U.S. Environmental Protection Agency
EQI	University of North Carolina-Ashville Environmental Quality Institute
FDA	U.S. Food and Drug Administration
FOIA	Freedom of Information Act
GAO	General Accounting Office
HEPA	High-efficiency particulate air (filter)
HHS	U.S. Department of Health and Human Services
HMO	Health Maintenance Organization
HUD	U.S. Department of Housing and Urban Development
IBWA	International Bottled Water Association
IG	Inspector General
IRS	Internal Revenue Service
LCCA	Lead Contamination Control Act
LIA	Lead Industries Association
NHANES II	Second National Health and Nutrition Examination Survey
NIOSH	National Institute for Occupational Safety and Health
NRDC	Natural Resources Defense Council
OSHA	Occupational Safety and Health Administration
PHS	U.S. Public Health Service
RCRA	Resource Conservation and Recovery Act
TRI	Toxic Release Inventory
TSP	Tri-Sodium Phosphate

APPENDIX B

LEAD INFORMATION HOTLINES AND RESOURCES

GENERAL

Alliance To End Childhood Lead Poisoning
227 Massachusetts Avenue NE, Suite 200
Washington, DC 20002
1-202-543-1147

Centers for Disease Control and Prevention
Lead Poisoning Prevention Branch
4770 Buford Highway NE
Building 101, mail drop 742
Atlanta, GA 30341
1-800-488-7330

Center for Safety in the Arts
5 Beekman Street, Suite 1030
New York, NY 10038
1-212-227-6220

National Lead Information Center
1-19 19th Street NW
Suite 401
Washington, DC 20036
(runs the following two hotlines)

National Lead Information Center
(General information for the public)
1-800-LEAD-FYI (1-800-532-3394)

National Lead Clearinghouse
(Technical information for professionals)
1-800-424-LEAD (1-800-424-5323)

National Maternal and Child Health Clearinghouse
1-703-821-8955

Western Regional Lead Training Consortium (WRLTC)
(States of Alaska, Arizona, California, Hawaii, Idaho, Nevada, Oregon, Washington)
1-800-572-LEAD (1-800-572-5323)

HOUSING

Department of Housing and Urban Development
Office of Lead Poisoning Prevention
451 7th Street SW (Room B-133)
Washington, DC 20410
Attn: Office of Lead Based Paint Abatement & Poison Prevention
1-800-245-2691

National Center for Lead-Safe Housing
1-410-992-0712

TOY RECALLS

Consumer Product Safety Commission
1-800-638-CPSC (1-800-638-2772)
  Teletypewriter for the hearing
  impaired,
(Outside Maryland): 1-800-638-8270
(Maryland only): 1-800-492-8104

WATER

EPA's Safe Drinking Water Hotline
1-800-426-4791

**International Bottled Water Association
  Hotline**
1-800-WATER-11 (1-800-928-3711)

WORK

**OSHA—U.S. Occupational Safety and
  Health Administration**
1-212-337-2378

National Lead Abatement Council
P.O. Box 535
Olney, MD 20832
1-301-924-0804

ADVOCATES

**Alliance To End Childhood Lead
  Poisoning**
600 Pennsylvania Avenue SE
Suite 100
Washington, DC 20003
1-202-543-1147

Conservation Law Foundation
62 Summer Street
Boston, MA 02110
1-617-350-0990

Environmental Defense Fund
257 Park Avenue South
New York, NY 10010
1-212-505-2100

Environmental Defense Fund
1875 Connecticut Avenue NW
Washington, DC 20009
1-202-387-3500

Natural Resources Defense Council
40 West 20th Street
New York, NY 10011
1-212-727-2700

APPENDIX C

MAIL-ORDER WATER TESTING

There are any number of laboratories which offer mail-order kits to test water for lead.

The following commercial labs all charge $35 for a first draw and flush lead-in-drinking-water test.

Water Test Corporation
33 S. Commercial Street
Manchester, NH 03101
1-800-426-8378

National Testing Laboratories
6151 Wilson Mills Road
Cleveland, OH 44143
1-800-458-3330

Suburban Water Testing Laboratories
4600 Kutztown Road
Temple, PA 19560
1-800-443-6595

EQI lab test kits are distributed by:

Clean Water Lead Testing
29½ Page Avenue
Asheville, NC 28801
($17.00/kit, includes S&H)

SAVE
P.O. Box 1723
FDR Station
New York, NY 10150
1-718-626-3936
($15.00/kit, plus $1.50/kit S&H)

Environmental Law Foundation
1736 Franklin Street, 7th Floor
Oakland, CA 94612
1-510-208-4555
($15.00/kit, plus flat $1.50 S&H)

APPENDIX D

STATE CONTACTS FOR ADDITIONAL INFORMATION ON LEAD

Alabama (205) 242-5766
Donna Hanes or Anic Lopez, R.N.
Childhood Lead Poisoning Prevention
Dr. Charles Woernle (205) 242-5131

Alaska (907) 790-2169
Linda Himmelbauer
Environmental Conservation
   Department

Arizona (602) 230-5861
Cecile Fowler
Screening and Lead Activities

Arkansas (501) 661-2592
Patsy Lewis or Dr. Bob West
Department of Health

California (510) 450-2453
L. Rex Ehling, Branch Chief
Childhood Lead Poisoning Prevention
Stephanie Gilmore
Public Outreach

Colorado (303) 692-2636
Amy Johnson
Department of Health
Michelle Bolyard (303) 692-3539
Water Quality Control Division

Connecticut (203) 566-5808
Narda Tolentino
Environmental Health Services

Delaware (302) 739-4735
Lisa Marencin
Special Health Needs Children

   WILMINGTON (302) 995-8693
Childhood Lead Poisoning Prevention

District of Columbia (202) 727-9870
Ella Witherspoon
Childhood Lead Poisoning Prevention

Florida (904) 488-3385
Roger Inman or Joseph Sekerke
State Health Office
Anne Boone (904) 488-9228
Medicaid Program

   PINELLAS COUNTY (813) 823-0401
Melanie Thoenes

Georgia (404) 657-6534
Ms. Tommie Bradford
Lead Poisoning Prevention Program

   FULTON COUNTY (404) 730-1491
Dr. Levonne Painter

Hawaii (808) 733-9022
Loretta Fuddy
Department of Health

Idaho (288) 334-6584
Steve West
Environmental Health

   PANHANDLE HEALTH DISTRICT
Jerry Cobb (208) 752-1235

Illinois 1-800-545-2200
Melinda Lehnherr or Jonah Deppe
Illinois Department of Public Health
(also) (217) 782-0403

KANKAKEE COUNTY (815) 937-7866
Val Messier
Health Department
Janice Marshall (815) 937-3565
Childhood Lead Poisoning Prevention

Indiana (317) 633-0662
David Ellsworth
Childhood Lead Poisoning Prevention
    Program

Iowa 1-800-972-2026
Ken Choquette (515) 282-8220
Rita Gergely (515) 242-6340
Childhood Lead Poisoning Prevention

Kansas
Steve Paige (913) 296-0189
Dick Morrissey (913) 296-1343
Dr. Andrew Pelletier (913) 296-5586
Dr. Dorothy Feese (913) 296-0688
Environmental Health Services

Kentucky (502) 564-2154
Ann Johnson, Sarah Wilding, or Pat
    Schmidt

NORTHERN KENTUCKY (606) 291-0770
Bill Bookmeyer or Cathy Winston
    (606) 491-6611
LEXINGTON/FAYETTE (606) 288-2434
Zaida Belendez, Carol Vaughn, or Carla
    Cornett
LOUISVILLE/JEFFERSON (502) 625-
    6648
Judy Nielsen or Connie Huber

Louisiana (504) 568-5070
Eve Flood
Office of Public Health

Maine (207) 287-3259
Edna Jones
Public Health Nursing
David Breau (207) 287-5694
Drinking Water

Maryland (410) 631-3859
Childhood Lead Poisoning Prevention
    Program

Massachusetts 1-800-532-9571
Jill Antonellis

MERRIMACK VALLEY (508) 681-4940
William O'Donnell
WORCESTER (508) 799-8589
Frank Birch
SOUTHEASTERN MASSACHUSETTS
    UNIVERSITY (508) 999-9930
Carmen Maiocco
BOSTON (617) 534-5965
Public Information Officer
SPRINGFIELD (413) 787-6717
Dolores Williams, Ph.D.
SALEM HOSPITAL (508) 745-2100
Ronna Fried-Lipsky, Ed.D.
LOWELL (508) 970-2470
Joan Seeler
AVON (508) 584-1414
Frances Olson
BARNSTABLE (508) 362-2511
Sean O'Brien

Michigan
LANSING (517) 335-8892
Alethia Carr
Lead Program Coordinator
Paulette Dunbar
    EPSDT/Lead Section Coordinator
Jim Bedford (517) 335-9215
Environmental Health (Abatement)
DETROIT (313) 876-4212
Harriett Billingslea
Childhood Lead Poisoning Control

Minnesota (612) 627-5017
Douglas Benson
Lead Program
Dianne Kocourek Ploetz (612) 627-5018

CITY OF ST. PAUL (612) 292-7747
Department of Health
Lynn Bahta
CITY OF MINNEAPOLIS (612) 673-3595
Brian Olson
Lead Program Coordinator

Mississippi (601) 960-7463
Ernest Griffin
Child Health Division

Missouri 1-800-392-7245
William Schmidt, Daryl Roberts, or
  Richard Gnaedinger
Department of Health
Kenneth Duzan (314) 751-7834
Missouri Department of Natural
  Resources

Montana (406) 444-3986
Todd Damerow
Health and Environmental Sciences

Nebraska (402) 471-0197
Rita Westover Medical Questions
Maternal and Child Health Division
Dr. Adi Pour (402) 471-2541
Bureau of Environmental Health

Nevada (702) 687-5240
David Going
Division of Enforcement for Safety

New Hampshire (603) 271-4507
Martha Turner Wells
Childhood Lead Poisoning Prevention
George Robinson (603) 271-4668
Public Health Laboratories
Todd Leedburg (603) 271-2942
Hazardous Waste Section
Richard Thayer Jr. (603) 271-3139
Environmental Services

  CITY OF MANCHESTER (603) 624-6466

New Jersey (609) 292-5666
Kevin McNally
State Department of Health
Danuta Budzygan (609) 588-2739
Medicaid Program, EPSDT
Bob Tucker (609) 984-6070
Department of Science and Research

  BURLINGTON COUNTY (609) 267-1950
  ext. 2832
Harriet Steuart
  CAMDEN COUNTY (609) 757-0021
John Costello
  CUMBERLAND COUNTY (609) 794-4264
Laurie Geremia, R.N.
  ESSEX COUNTY
East Orange (201) 266-5489
Irvington (201) 399-6651
Newark (201) 733-7547 or 456-5032
Orange (201) 266-4077
  GLOUCESTER COUNTY (609) 853-3437
Delle Zelinsky
  HUDSON COUNTY (201) 547-4567
Madeline Brown
  MIDDLESEX COUNTY (908) 521-1402
Joan Pisuk
Nina Benton (908) 745-6663
  MONMOUTH/OCEAN COUNTY (908)
  431-7456
Jeryl Krautle
Theresa Comfroy (908) 341-9700
  PASSAIC COUNTY (201) 881-6919
Majorie Pacheco
  TRENTON (609) 989-3204
Sharon Winn
  UNION COUNTY (908) 289-8600
Barbara Parker
Imelda Chukwu (908) 753-3500

New Mexico (505) 827-0006
Dan Merians
Epidemiology

New York (518) 473-4602
Nancy Robinson, James Raucci, or
  Marie Miller
Bureau of Child and Adolescent Health
Patrick Parsons (518) 474-5475
Center for Laboratories and Research

  WESTCHESTER COUNTY (914) 593-
  5203
Donna Bernard
  NEW YORK CITY (212) BAN-LEAD
Lead Poisoning Prevention Program
Water Test, NYDEP (718) 699-9811
Department of Housing, Preservation
  and Development (212) 960-4800

North Carolina
Ed Normans (919) 733-0385
Division of Maternal and Child Health
James Hayes (919) 733-2884
Environmental Health Services

North Dakota (701) 224-2493
David Cunningham or Sandra Anseth
Childhood Lead Poisoning Prevention
Ken Kary (701) 221-2169
Mike Borr (701) 221-6143
Public Health Laboratories
Dana Mount or Ken Wangler (701) 221-5188
Environmental Services

Ohio (614) 466-5332
Darlene Baney
Lead Program Coordinator
Phil Hyde (614) 644-1894
Environmental Health

CLEVELAND (216) 664-2175
Wayne Slota
COLUMBUS (614) 645-6129
Gary Garver
MAHONING COUNTY (216) 788-7571
Karla Krodel
CINCINNATI (513) 352-3052
Shirley Wilkinson

Oklahoma (405) 271-4471
Dr. Edd Rhoades
Medical Questions, Maternal and Child Health
Monty Elder (405) 271-7353
Environmental Questions

Oregon (503) 731-4000
Oregon Health Division

Pennsylvania
Contact your local state health center.
Lead Poisoning Programs:

ALLEGHENY (412) 823-3120
N.E. PENNSYLVANIA 1-800-662-5220
HARRISBURG (717) 782-2884

Rhode Island (401) 277-3424
Peter Simon, M.D., MPH,
Family Health
Cathy O'Malley (401) 277-2312
Childhood Lead Poisoning Control

South Carolina
COLUMBIA (803) 737-4061
Pam Meyer or Charlotte McCreary
Children's Health Division
CHARLESTON (803) 724-5891
Jackie Dawson
Lead Poisoning

South Dakota (605) 773-3364
Kevin Forsch
Health Protection

Tennessee (615) 741-5683
Dr. Robert Taylor
Environmental Epidemiology

Texas 1-800-422-2956
GALVESTON (409) 772-1561
Wayne R. Snodgrass, M.D.
DALLAS (214) 670-7151
Alice Pita, M.D.
SAN ANTONIO (512) 270-3971
Dr. Michael Foulds, M.D.
HOUSTON
Dr. Marcus Hanfling (713) 793-2592
Sonja A. Vodehnal, MPA (713) 794-9349

Utah (801) 538-6191
Dr. Denise Beaudoin
Medical Questions, Epidemiological Studies Program
Daniel Symonik (801) 536-4171
Environmental Questions
Wayne Pierce (801) 584-8400
Laboratory Testing Questions

Vermont 1-800-439-8550
Karen Garbarino (802) 865-7786
Childhood Lead Poisoning Prevention Program

Virginia 1-800-523-4019
Eileen M. Mannix (804) 786-7367
Maternal and Child Health Division
Edward Lefebvre (804) 786-3766
Consolidated Laboratory Services
 Division
Jack Proctor (804) 786-5041
Building Regulatory Services

 CENTRAL VIRGINIA (804) 947-6777
Dr. Edward Hancock
 CRATER HEALTH DISTRICT (804) 861-
 6582
Daphne Homer
 NORFOLK HEALTH DISTRICT (804)
 683-2862
Kris Meek
 PORTSMOUTH HEALTH DISTRICT (804)
 393-8585
Susan Strong, R.N. (ext. 152)
RICHMOND HEALTH DISTRICT (804) 780-
 4240
Yvonne Johnson
 FAIRFAX COUNTY (703) 246-2411

Washington (206) 753-2730
David F. Nash
Department of Health

West Virginia (304) 558-0197
Cathy Hayes
Office of Laboratory Sciences

Wisconsin
Mark Chamberlain (608) 266-7897
Abatement
Jody Diedrich (608) 266-1826
Medical
Joe Schirmer (608) 266-5885
General
Patty Bolig (608) 266-5817
Laboratory

 CITY OF MILWAUKEE (414) 225-LEAD

Wyoming (307) 777-7957
Howard Hutchings
Environmental Health Program

Source: Environmental Health Center of the National Safety Council

APPENDIX E

HUD REGIONAL OFFICES

HUD REGION	ADDRESS/PHONE
1	Boston Regional Office Room 375 Thomas P. O'Neill, Jr. Federal Building 10 Causeway Street Boston, MA 02222-1092 (617) 565-5234
2	New York Regional Office 26 Federal Plaza New York, NY 10278-0068 (212) 264-6500
3	Philadelphia Regional Office Liberty Square Building 105 South Seventh Street Philadelphia, PA 19106-3392 (215) 597-2560
4	Atlanta Regional Office Richard B. Russell Federal Building 75 Spring Street SW Atlanta, GA 30303-3388 (404) 331-5138
5	Chicago Regional Office Ralph Metcalfe Federal Building 77 West Jackson Boulevard Chicago, IL 60604-3507 (312) 353-5680

6

Fort Worth Regional Office
1600 Throckmorton
P.O. Box 2905
Fort Worth, TX 76113-2905
(817) 885-5401

7

Kansas City Regional Office
Room 200 Gateway Tower II
400 State Avenue
Kansas City, KS 66101-2400
(913) 236-2162

8

Denver Regional Office
Executive Tower Building
1405 Curtis Street
Denver, CO 80202-2349
(303) 844-4513

9

San Francisco Regional Office
Philip Burton Federal Building
450 Golden Gate Avenue
P.O. Box 36003
San Francisco, CA 94102-3448
(415) 556-4752

Indian Programs Office
Suite 1650
2 Arizona Center
400 North Fifth Street
Phoenix, AZ 85004-2361
(602) 379-4156

10

Seattle Regional Office
Arcade Plaza Building
1321 Second Avenue
Seattle, WA 96101-2058
(206) 553-5414

APPENDIX F

EPA REGIONAL OFFICES

EPA REGION	CONTACT
1	Ann Carroll JFK Federal Building One Congress Street Boston, MA 02203 (617) 565-3411 (617) 565-3415 (Fax)
2	Lou Bevilacqua Building 5, SDPTSB 2890 Woodbridge Avenue Edison, NJ 08837-3679 (908) 321-6671 (908) 321-6757 (Fax)
3	Fran Dougherty 841 Chestnut Building Philadelphia, PA 19107 (215) 597-8322 (215) 597-7906 (Fax)
4	Connie Landers 345 Courtland Street NE Atlanta, GA 30365 (404) 347-1033 (404) 347-1681 (Fax)
5	David Turpin SP-14J 77 West Jackson Street Chicago, IL 60604 (312) 886-7836 (312) 353-4342 (Fax)

6

Jeff Robinson
12th Floor, Suite 2000
1445 Ross Avenue
Dallas, TX 75202
(214) 655-7577
(214) 655-2164 (Fax)

7

Mazzie Talley
726 Minnesota Avenue
Kansas City, KA 66101
(913) 551-7518
(913) 551-7065 (Fax)

8

David Combs
999 18th Street
Suite 500
Denver, CO 80202
(303) 293-1442
(303) 293-1488 (Fax)

9

Jo Ann Semones
75 Hawthorne Street
San Francisco, CA 94105
(415) 744-1128
(415) 744-1073 (Fax)

10

Barbara Ross
Toxics Section
1200 Sixth Avenue
Seattle, WA 98101
(206) 553-1985
(206) 553-8338 (Fax)

APPENDIX G

LINERS AND ENCAPSULANTS

BRAND NAME	MANUFACTURER	OVERCOAT WITH:
CANVAS WALL LINERS		
Sanitas Lining	GenCorp 3 University Plaza #200 Hackensack, NJ 07601 (201) 489-0100	Paint or paper
Wall-Tex Lining Canvas	Sunwall of America 2925 Courtyards Drive Norcross, GA 30071 1-800-523-8006	Paint or paper
POLYESTER WALL LINERS		
BRIDGEALL Wall Lining	GenCorp	Paper
Fashion UNDERCOVER	GenCorp	Paper
Essex Wallcoverings VINYLINER	GenCorp	Paper
Cover-Ups	Sunwall of America	Paint or paper
Home Wall Prepasted Wall Liner	Patton Wall Coverings P.O. Box 12002 Columbus, OH 43212 1-800-848-1488	Paper
Heavy Duty Wall Liner	Patton Wall Coverings	Paint or paper
R. M. Wall	R. M. Inc. 4039 West Green Tree Road Milwaukee, WI 53209 1-800-558-0434	Paper

FIBERGLASS WALL LINERS

OLID-WALL   The Glidden Company   Paint or paper
925 Euclid Avenue
Cleveland, OH 44115
1-800-221-4100

Nu-Wal   Specification Chemicals   Paint or paper
824 Keeler Street
Boone, IA 50036
1-800-247-3932

LIQUID ENCAPSULANT SOURCES

BRAND NAME	MANUFACTURER
AGP Protecta- Poxy Series 200EC	AGP Surfaces Control Systems (518) 734-5880
ASTEC #100	Advance Coating and Spray Inc. (412) 486-0295
CTI Series	CTI (Concrete Technology Inc.) (813) 535-4651
Certane 4000, 4050	Certech (Certified Technologies Corporation) 1-800-433-1892
First Coat Mirrolac WB Pre Prime 167	Devoe and Reynolds Company (502) 589-9340
Back to Nature Safe Encapsulant	Dynacraft Industries (908) 303-8920
Elite-Cap	Elite Coatings Company (912) 628-2111
Encapseal Encap Mesh	Encap Systems Corporation 1-800-732-9156
Encapsulastic 7000 (Trim and Exterior) Encapsulastic 8000 (Walls and Ceilings)	Encapsulation Corporation (410) 962-5335

Wall Coating Ceiling Coat Trim Coating	Fiber Tec Coatings Corporation (704) 841-8527
FX-499 Hydro-Ester Coating or Mortar	Fox Industries (410) 243-8856
Saf-T-Seal ArmaGlaze (A & B)	I.C., Inc. (410) 252-5650
Lead Seal	International Protective Coatings Corporation (908) 531-3666
Kapsulkote	Kapsulkote Inc. 1-800-328-5885
Lead Block 3000 Good Advice Primer	Premier Coatings Inc. (708) 439-4200
Saf-T-Shield LBP Encapsulation Coatings	Proko Industries 1-800-423-8341
Cover-up Cover-all Radox (Lead-Tec)	Mateson Chemical Corporation 1-800-434-0010

Courtesy Maryland Department of the Environment

APPENDIX H

HOME LEAD TEST KITS

Consumer Reports recently examined the two test kits listed below and noted what the kits can do and what they can't do. The observations generally hold for all in-home do-it-yourself lead-test kits:

- They're inexpensive and produce results quickly.
- The readings are not very precise.
- They only tell whether the sample contains some lead; neither kit can tell you how much lead is present.
- Neither kit is sensitive to low levels of lead, so some items that test negative may not be completely safe.

Kits tested by *Consumer Reports:*

Leadcheck Swabs, available from:

> HybriVet Systems, Inc.
> P.O. Box 1210
> Framingham, MA 01701
> 1-800-262-LEAD
> Price: $23.95 plus shipping, for 12 test swabs
> *Leadcheck Swabs* can often be found in local hardware stores and through home catalogs.

Frandon Lead Alert Kit, available from:

> Frandon Enterprises
> 511 North 48th
> Seattle, WA 98103
> 1-800-359-9000 to order (Mastercard/Visa)
> Price: $19.95 plus shipping, for 40 tests
> $29.95 plus shipping, for 100 tests

Other lead-test kits, not tested by *Consumer Reports,* include:

Lead Inspector Kit, available from:

> Michigan Ceramic Supply Inc.
> 4048 Seventh Street
> P.O. Box 342

Wyandotte, MI 48192
(313) 281-2300
Price: $17.95 plus shipping, for 100 tests

The Lead Detective, available from:

Innovative Synthesis Corporation
45 Lexington Street, Suite 2
Newton, MA 02165
(617) 244-9078
Price: $29.95 plus shipping, for 100 tests

All of these products can be used to detect high levels of lead in ceramics, paint, and solder.

APPENDIX I

TOY RECALLS

The following toys have been recalled by the Consumer Product Safety Commission (CPSC) over the past three years for violations of the law banning lead-in-paint on children's toys.

PRODUCT	MANUFACTURER
Butterfly Puzzle #MTC-2030	Animal Quacker Ltd.
Garden Tools Puzzle #MTC-2028	Greensboro, NC
Rooster Puzzle #MTC-2033	
Snail Puzzle #MTC-2032	
Table Setting Puzzle #MTC-2029	
Tool Puzzle #MTC-2027	
Turtle Puzzle #MTC-2031	
Vegetable Puzzle #MTC-2026	
Hanging Checkerboard #0Q099	Cape Shore, Inc.
Hanging Checkerboard #00099	Yarmouth, ME
Colortone Eight Crayon Box #5-CL-850	Dynamic Stationery Manufacturing Hollis, NY
Busy Farm Trucks #448-09883	Fast Rolling Books
Busy School Bus #448-09880	Zokeisha (USA) Ltd.
Fast Rolling Fire Trucks #448-09876	New York, NY
Fast Rolling Little Engine #448-09878	
Fast Rolling Work Trucks #448-09877	
Santa's Sleigh #448-10282	
Tough Trucks #448-09884	
Abribois Paint—Ripolin-1	Fine Paints of France
Abrifer Paint—Ripolin-1	Grove, NY
500 Superlaque Brilliant—Ripolin-1	

500 Superlaque Satine—Ripolin-l
  Blooming
Vernis Ebenisterie—Ripolin-1
Vernis Yachting Paint—Ripolin-1

Air Time Pogo Stick #7730	GPT Products Elmhurst, IL

Baby Bop backpacks and carry-all
  bags
Barney backpacks and carry-all
  bags
vinyl beach bags (three styles)
	Jaclyn, Inc.
	West New York, NJ

Slinky Toy #440 Frog Slinky Toy #480 Kitten Slinky Toy #425 Seal Slinky Toy #200 Train Slinky Toy #250 Worm	James Industries, Inc. Hollidayburg, PA

Mandarin Chair #39A-Y Grey
Mandarin Chair #39A-5 Red
Spyder Table #3ZTRI-G1/2-1 6-
  Y Grey
Spyder Table #3ZTRI-G1/2-1 6-5
  Red
	Knoll International, Inc.
	East Greenville, PA

electric toy train #8113 electric toy train #8506	Life-Like Products, Inc. Baltimore, MD
Chubby Children's Paint Brush Set #220, LV-4853 water color and brushes #LV8888	Lillian Vernon Corporation Mt. Vernon, NY
Crib Center #1525 Pull Along Loco #T105002	Little Tikes Co. Hudson, OH
Paint Brushes—Do It Yourself	Marx Brush Mfg. Company Palisades Park, NJ
mops, brooms, sticks	Nu-Cushion Product Manufacturing Company Shawnee Mission, KA
Fashion Flair-10 oz. Spray Paint	Plasti-Kote Company, Inc. Medina, OH
Jumpin' Jeans Denim Paint Kits Paint Brush in Various Kits	Polymerics, Inc.-Tulip Prods. Waltham, MA
Thunder Max 2000 Ride-On Toy #4031	SLM Gloversville, NY

Putt-Putt Orange Paint #12432	Southern Gold Distributors Fayetteville, NC
Activity Rocker #390 Kids Workbench #690 Super Car #1050	Today's Kids Booneville, AR
Music Master Xylophone #SX- 305—SKN 421944	Toys "R" Us Paramus, NJ
Plastercraft #7440	Tyco Industries, Inc. Mt. Laurel, NJ

The following crayons, imported from China, were recalled in 1994 by the CPSC because of high lead content (one child was known to be poisoned by them):

PRODUCT	MANUFACTURER
64 Crayons, School Quality, No. 8064	A.J. Cohen Distributors Hauppauge, NY
64 Crayons, Kidz Biz	Bargain Wholesale Los Angeles, CA
64 Crayons, #CR 64-64 CT	Baum Imports New York, NY
12 Jumbo Crayons	Concord Enterprises Los Angeles, CA
8 Crayons, No. 5 CL 850 12 Super Jumbo Crayons and	Dynamic Division of Agora International St. Albans, NY
12 Crayons, Glory and 18 Crayons That Paint	Glory Stationery Manufacturing Company, Ltd. Los Angeles, CA
Feido, 12 Crayons, No. CC8812	Kipp Brothers Inc. Indianapolis, IN
Fun Time 72 Crayons, No. B541	Overseas United New York, NY
Safe 48 Non-Toxic I'm a Toys "R" Us Kid! Crayons	Toys "R" Us Paramus, NJ
64 Crayons, SKU#51-02600	Universal International Minneapolis, MN

After the Food and Drug Administration detected excessive lead levels in samplings of these tea and dishware sets, the following products were recalled by their distributors, Chilton-Globe, Inc., of Manitowoc, Wisconsin; Friendly Home Parties, Inc., of Albany, New York; McCrory Corp. of York, Pennsylvania; and Lillian Vernon Corp. of Mount Vernon, New York:

Barbie China Dinner Set (16 pieces)	Product #3338-9
Barbie China 12-Piece Tea Set	Product #3334-9
Cabbage Patch Kids China Set (13 pieces)	Product #3346-9
Campbell's 15-Piece Soup Time China Set	Product #3351-9
Campbell's 9-Piece Soup Time China Set	Product #3350-9
Children's China Tea Set	Product #832543
Chilton Toys 12-Piece Tea Set	Product #3331-9
Friendly Home Parties Porcelain Tea Set	Catalogue #323
Holly Hobbie China Dinner Set (16 pieces)	Product #3340-9
Holly Hobbie China Tea Set (12 pieces)	Product #3339-9
Porcelain Tea Set for Children	Catalogue #482589

APPENDIX J

UNSAFE WATER COOLERS

WATER COOLERS WITH LEAD-LINED TANKS

The following list of model numbers represents all of the drinking-water coolers with lead-lined tanks that have been identified and reported on by the EPA. The models listed here were selected because one or more of the units in that model series have been tested and found to have lead-lined tanks.

Halsey Taylor Company:

WM 8A	GC 10A
WT 8A	GC 5A
GC 10ACR	RWM 13A

OTHER WATER COOLERS CONTAINING LEAD

Halsey Taylor Company:

WMA-1	SCWT/SCWT-A
SWA-1	DC/DHC-1
S3/5/10D	BFC-4F/7F/4FS/7FS
S300/500/1000D	

In addition to these Halsey Taylor models, Halsey Taylor indicates that the following Haws brand coolers manufactured for Haws by Halsey Taylor from November 1984, through December 18, 1987, are not lead free because they contain two tin-lead solder joints. The model designations for these coolers are:

HC8WT	HC14W	HCBF7D
HC8WTH	HC4F	HCBF7HO
HC14WT	HC4FH	HWC7
HC14WTH	HC8F	HWC7D
HC14WL	HC8FH	HC2F
HC16WT	HC14F	HC2FH

HC4W	HC14FH	HC5F
HC6W	HC14FL	HC10F
HC8W	HCBF7	

EBCO Manufacturing Company:

EBCO has identified all pressure bubbler water coolers with shipping dates from 1962 through 1977 as having a bubbler valve containing lead, as defined by the LCCA. The units contain a single 50-50 tin-lead solder joint on the bubbler valve. Model numbers for those coolers in this category were not available.

The following EBCO models of pressure bubbler coolers produced from 1978 through 1981 contain one 50-50 tin-lead solder joint each:

CP3	DP7SM	DPM8H
CP10-50	DP10F	DP16M
DP20-50	CP3H	DP7S
DP13A	13P	DP7WM
DP7M	DP3RH	EP10F
DP13M-60	DP14A-50/60	CP10
CP5M	DP12N	DP20
DP14S	DPM8	DP8AH
DP5F	DP15M	C10E
CP3-50	DP5S	DP5M
7P	DP13SM	DP13M
DP3R	EP5F	CP3M
DP13A-50	CP5	DP13S
PX-10	13PL	DP7WMD
DP7MH	DP8A	WTC10
DP14M	DP10X	
DP15MW	DP15W	

Pressure bubbler water coolers manufactured by EBCO and marketed under the brand names Oasis and Kelvinator with the identified model numbers have also been distributed in the United States. EBCO indicated that Aquarius pressure bubbler water coolers are manufactured for distribution in foreign countries, including Canada. Although unlikely, it is conceivable that an Aquarius cooler with one of the model numbers listed above could have been transported into the United States.

APPENDIX K

SAMPLE FREEDOM OF INFORMATION REQUEST

A Freedom of Information request to your regional EPA office can get you information about contamination (including but not limited to lead) on or near your property or in your community. EPA maintains several data bases with this information. One, called CERCLIS, is part of the national Superfund program and lists all potentially contaminated sites. The other, called the Toxic Release Inventory, or TRI, lists companies that have released contaminated substances into the local environment.

To get information for your locality, you may need to make two requests. The first is a general request for any information about possible sites near where you live or where you may be considering moving. A sample letter:

FOIA Officer
U.S. Environmental Protection Agency
(Insert local address for your region.
See appendix F.)

Dear FOIA Officer,

This is a formal request under the Freedom of Information Act (FOIA) for a CERCLIS printout of both active and inactive hazardous waste sites for (insert your town or county and state). Please also include any TRI data for this locality. Please send the information to (insert your name and address).

If there is a charge for this printout, please contact me at (insert your phone number).

Thank you for your cooperation.

Very truly yours,

The result of this request will be a list of toxic material releases, plus any contaminated sites that may be in your area. Should there be potentially contaminated sites, you can get more specific information about what types of contamination may be present. To do that, you will need to submit a second letter:

FOIA Officer
U.S. Environmental Protection Agency
(Insert local address for your region.
See appendix F.)

Dear FOIA Officer,

This is a formal request under the Freedom of Information Act (FOIA) to review the USEPA files for (insert number of sites) that are listed on the Comprehensive Environmental Liability, Response and Compensation List (CERCLIS) data base maintained by the USEPA. The properties are:

(Insert site information as it appeared on the list obtained as a result of your first letter, i.e.:

NJD001396985
FMC Corporation Special Products Group
326 South Dean Street
Englewood, NJ 07631)

Please send the information to (insert your name and address). If there is a charge for this printout, please contact me at (insert your phone number).

Thank you for your cooperation.

Very truly yours,

APPENDIX L

LEAD ABATEMENT TRAINING CENTERS

These training centers are run through a cooperative agreement between the EPA and the National University Continuing Education Association. The centers provide training in lead inspection and abatement activities. The address and phone number for each center are listed below:

Northeast Regional Lead Training
   Center
School of Public Health
Public Health Building
University of Massachusetts, Amherst
Amherst, MA 01003
(413) 545-4222

Mideastern and Atlantic Regional Lead
   Training Center (Maryland)
School of Medicine
University of Maryland, Baltimore
28 East Ostland Street
Baltimore, MD 21230
(410) 706-1849

Southern Regional Lead Training Center
Georgia Tech Research Institute
Environmental Science and Technology
   Laboratory
Atlanta, GA 30332
(404) 894-3806

Mideastern and Atlantic Regional Lead
   Training Center (Cincinnati)
Department of Environmental Health
University of Cincinnati
3223 Eden Avenue, ML-0056
Cincinnati, OH 45267-0056
(513) 558-1729

Midwestern Regional Lead Training
   Center
Division of Continuing Education
University of Kansas
P.O. Box 25936
Overland Park, KS 66225-4936
(913) 897-8500

Western Regional Lead Training Center
15090 Avenue of Science
Suite 103
San Diego, CA 92128
(619) 451-7460
1-800-572-LEAD (available only to
   people living in Alaska, Arizona,
   California, Hawaii, Idaho, Nevada,
   Oregon, and Washington)

APPENDIX M

CHRONOLOGY OF
RECENT LEAD LEGISLATION

1970   The United States Congress begins taking action to address lead poisoning under the Clean Air Act of 1970.

1971   The phaseout of leaded gasoline begins.

Congress passes the Lead-Based Paint Poisoning Prevention Act, which is a national effort to identify children with lead poisoning and abate the sources of lead in their environments.

1976   Under the Resource Conservation and Recovery Act (RCRA), lead is classified as a hazardous waste if it leaches into the ground at concentrations above 5 parts per million and therefore becomes subject to detailed removal and disposal requirements.

1978   National Ambient Air Quality Standards (NAAQS) are set for lead at 1.5 micrograms per cubic meter of air ($\mu g/m^3$).

1980   Comprehensive Environmental Response, Compensation, and Liability Act (Superfund) was enacted. Although there are no specific provisions for lead, three cities have received Superfund monies to carry out soil-lead abatement demonstration projects to remove the long-term deposits of lead in soils.

1986   The Superfund Amendments and Reauthorization Act (SARA) Toxic Release Inventory (TRI) requires certain industrial sources of lead to report their annual releases to the environment.

1988   The Lead Contamination Control Act appropriates monies to state and local governments to perform childhood lead screening, give medical referrals, and provide education about the risks associated with elevated blood lead levels.

1991   Research and evaluation programs for monitoring, detecting, and abating lead-based paint and other lead exposure hazards in housing and for other purposes were included in the Technology Preeminence Act of 1991.

1992   Title X of the Residential Housing and Community Development Act will require owners or landlords, of housing built before 1978, to inform prospective buyers or renters about known lead-based paint in the properties beginning in 1995. During that same year, rental property owners receiving government subsidies must inspect for and reduce lead contamination in buildings constructed before 1978. Federal agencies must also remove lead-based hazards in foreclosure properties built before 1960; otherwise the prospective buyer or renter must be informed about any lead-based hazards.

INDEX

Page numbers in italics refer to boxed text.

Kashtock, Michael, 112
Kennedy Krieger Institute, 29, 32, 51, 68, 180
Kessler, David A., 118

Labeling of Hazardous Art Materials Act, 146
Landlord(s), 51, 55, 68
and abatement, 181–82
Landlord liability, 172–74
Lantos, Tom, 176–77
Laws/legislation
chronology of, 215–16
control of lead exposure, 182–83
lead abatement, 180–83
lead-based paint in housing, 169, 170, 172
Lawsuits, 173–74, 181
Leaching, 85, 90, 94, 103, 171
from crystal, 116–17
in dishes, 107, 108, 109, 110, 112, 115, 143
from faucets, 85–89
in fruit juices, 106
rates of, 87
standards for china, 113, 114
from water coolers, 129
Lead
attacking body, 11–13
disposal of materials containing, 147–48
precautions in working with, 145–48
see also Dust, lead; Paint, lead
Lead acetate, 45
"Lead Based Paint—Protect Your Family" (booklet), 58
Lead-Based Poisoning Prevention Act, 37
Lead casting, 140, 144, 147, 158–59
Lead Contamination Control Act, 129
Lead Exposure Reduction Act (proposed), 82
Lead Free Faucets, Inc., 89
"Lead in School Drinking Water" (booklet), 130–31
Lead Industries Association (LIA), 36–37

Lead industry, 10, 36–37, 178–80, 185
Lead-pipe water systems, 2, 84–85, 93, 94, 95
Lead poisoning, xi–xii, 1–14, 16, 23–24, 184–85
basic facts about, 2–5
and criminality, 5, 10, 185
daily levels of lead ingestion resulting in, 12
from food and drink, 106–7
signs of, 5
see also Acute lead poisoning; Low-level lead poisoning; Symptoms
Lead poisoning classification, 21, 21–22, 24–29, 42, 50
"Lead Poisoning Prevention Act" (draft), 182–83
Lead poisoning programs, 18–19
Lead-risk assessor, 54, 57
Lead shot, 133–34, 160, 167–68
Lead sinkers, 157–59, 167
Lead-test kits, 1, 204–5
Lead vapors
see Fumes, lead
Learning disability(ies), xii, 1, 5, 16, 26
LEDIZOLV, 22, 65
Liability, 171
industry, 174–76
landlord, 172–74, 182
Lifetime Faucets, 88–89
Liners (list), 201–3
Locations outside the home
checking for hazards, 126–28
Low-level lead poisoning, 3–4, 40, 51, 52, 57, 156, 169, 179
from dishes, 110
effects of, 5
halting, 17

Maas, Richard P., 86–87, 88
Market-share damages, 175–76
Maryland, 33, 46, 62, 63, 68, 137
Division of Lead Poisoning Prevention, 64
lead abatement law, 180–83